Chambers

Medical
Spelling Checker

D1343951

Also published by Chambers

Spell Well
Type Right!
Chambers Pocket Guide to Good Spelling

Dr Elizabeth McCall-Smith is a general medical practitioner in Edinburgh

Chambers

Medical
Spelling Checker

Edited by

Dr Elizabeth McCall-Smith

Published by W & R Chambers Ltd Edinburgh, 1989

British Library Cataloguing in Publication Data

McCall-Smith, Elizabeth
   Chambers medical spelling checker.
   1. Medicine – Encyclopaedias
   I. Title
   610'.3'21

ISBN 0-550-18041-9

Cover design by William Ross Design
Typeset by Bookworm Typesetting Ltd, Edinburgh
Printed in Great Britain at the University Press, Cambridge

Preface

Good spelling is essential for everyone in the medical profession, whether they be doctor, dentist, nurse or medical secretary. It is rare, though, to find someone who can spell all the words they are called upon to type or write during the course of their working day. A general dictionary might not contain specialized medical vocabulary, and although a medical dictionary is useful, it is not always necessary to know the precise *meaning* of a word, but simply its spelling, in order to be able to transcribe accurately and quickly from a dictation or notes.

Chambers Medical Spelling Checker contains over 25,000 words clearly arranged in alphabetical order. It combines a large general vocabulary with medical terms and generic and approved trade names of drugs found in the British National Formulary. It thus avoids the need for two or more different reference sources. Word definitions have not been included, as the primary intention of the book is to facilitate the quick and easy checking of spelling.

Additional sections contain lists of degrees, diplomas and qualifications; commonly used units of measurement and how to type them; and common abbreviations.

In all, *Chambers Medical Spelling Checker* is a handy desktop reference.

About this book

The 25,000 words are clearly arranged in alphabetical order. In some instances there is more than one correct spelling for a word, and which spelling is used is a matter of individual preference. Alternative spellings are listed in the correct alphabetical position, and therefore the alternative spelling or a single word may not be listed consecutively.

For verb endings -ize rather -ise has used been consistently, and English rather than American spelling has been used throughout, as in haemoglobin, goitre, foetus.

All trade names have been marked with an ®, as in Actrapid® and Fungilin®.

Words which are not spelled the way they sound

Certain words might cause difficulty because they are not spelled the way they sound. In particular note the following:

the silent 'p' as in:

eg phimosis	(pronounced 'thimosos')
psoriasis	(pronounced 'soriasis')
pterygium	(pronounced 'terygium')
psychological	(pronounced 'sycological')
pneumonia	(pronounced 'neumonia')

some words pronounced with'V' begin with'W':

eg Wertheim	(pronounced 'vertheim')
Weber	(pronounced 'veber')
Wasserman	(pronounced 'vasserman')

'y' is often used for the sound 'i':

eg dysplasia	is pronounced 'displasia'
lymphatic	is pronounced 'limphatic'

Word division and word breaks

Where it has been necessary to divide a word, the division is indicated by a centred dot as in:

agamma·
globulinaemia

Commonsense and the overall appearance of the printed page are important considerations for end-of-line divisions.

If a word has to be split at the end of a line, the split should be between two syllables. The word should be divided according to its sound when speaking aloud so that its meaning is entirely clear to the reader.

A split should not divide a word so that a part of it, which is a word in its own right, is divided:

eg ketoacidosis should be divided keto-acidosis and not ketoacid-osis because acidosis is a word in its own right and ketoacid is not.

A single letter of a word should not begin or end a line.

Aa

aback
abacterial
abandon
abasement
abasia
abate
abated
abating
abattoir
abbreviate
abbreviated
abbreviating
abbreviation
abdicate
abdicated
abdicating
abdication
abdomen
abdominal
abdominocentesis
abdominoperineal
abducent
abduct
abduction
abductor
aberrant
aberration
abet
abetalipoproteinaemia
abetted
abetting
abeyance
abhor
abhorred
abhorrence
abhorrent
abhorring
abide by
Abidec®

abided by
abiding by
abilities
ability
ablation
able
ablutions
ably
abnormal
abnormalities
abnormality
abnormally
abode by
abolish
abolition
abominable
abort
abortifacient
abortion
abortive
abortus
abound
abrasion
abrasive
abreaction
abreast
abridge
abridged
abridging
abrupt
abruption
abruptio placentae
abscess
abscesses
abscissa
abscond
absence
absent
absentee
absolute
absolutely
absorb

absorbent
absorption
abstain
abstinence
abstract
abstraction
absurd
absurdities
absurdity
abundance
abundant
abuse
abused
abusing
abusive
abysmal
abysmally
academic
academically
academies
academy
acalulia
acanthocytosis
acantholysis
acanthoma
acanthosis
Acanthosis nigricans
Acari
acaricide
Acarus
accelerate
accelerated
accelerating
acceleration
accelerator
accent
accentuate
accentuated
accentuating
accept
acceptable
acceptance

access
accessibility
accessible
accessibly
accessories
accessory
accident
accidental
accidentally
acclimatization
acclimatize
acclimatized
acclimatizing
accommodate
accommodated
accommodating
accommodation
accommodative
accompanied
accompaniment
accompany
accompanying
accomplish
accord
accordance
according
accordingly
account
accountable
accountant
accredited
accretion
accumulate
accumulated
accumulating
accumulation
accuracy
accurate
accusation
accuse
accused
accuser

accusing
accustomed
acebutolol
ACE inhibitor
Acepril®
acetabula
acetabuloplasty
acetabulum
acetaldehyde
acetate
acetazolamide
acetic
acetic acid
aceto-acetate
acetohexamide
acetomenaphthone
acetone
acetonide
Acetoxyl®
acetylcholine
acetylcysteine
acetylene
Acezide®
achalasia
ache
ached
achieve
achieved
achievement
achieving
Achilles tendon
aching
achlorhydria
acholia
acholuria
acholuric
achondroplasia
achondroplastic
achromatopsia
Achromycin®
Achromycin V®
acid

acidaemia
acid-base balance
acid-fast
acidification
acidify
acidity
acidophil
acidophilic
acidosis
acid phosphatase
aciduria
Aci-Jel®
acinar
acini
acinous
acinus
acipimox
acknowledge
acknowledged
acknowledgement
acknowledging
acne
acneform
Acnegel®
acneiform
acne vulgaris
acoustic
acoustically
acoustic nerve
acoustics
acquaint
acquaintance
acquire
acquired
acquired immune
  deficiency
  syndrome
acquiring
acquisition
acquittal
acrocentric
acrocephalic

acrocephalous
acrocephaly
acrocyanosis
acrocyanotic
acrolein
acromegalic
acromegaly
acromial
acromioclavicular
acromion
acrosclerosis
acrosoxacin
across
acrylic
Actal®
Acthar Gel®
Actidil®
Actifed®
actin
Actinac®
actinic
Actinobacillus
Actinomyces
actinomycin D
actinomycosis
action
actionable
activate
activated
activating
activator
active
activities
activity
Actraphane®
Actrapid®
Actrapid Penfill®
actual
actually
acuity
Acupan®
acupuncture

acute
acyanosis
acyanotic
acyclovir
Adalat®
adamant
Adam's apple
adapt
adaptability
adaptable
Adcortyl®
addenda
addendum
adder
addict
addicted
addiction
addictive
Addison's disease
addition
additional
additionally
additive
address
addressed
addressee
addresses
addressing
adduct
adduction
adductor
adelomorphic
adenectomy
adenine
adenitis
adenocarcinoma
adenocarcinomata
adenocarcinomatous
adenocyte
adenoidectomy
adenoids
adenoma

adenomata
adenomatous
adenomyoma
adenomyomata
adenomyomatous
adenomyosis
adenopathy
adenosarcoma
adenosine
   diphosphate (ADP)
adenosine
   triphosphate (ATP)
adenovirus
adept
adequacy
adequate
adequately
adhere
adhered
adherence
adherent
adhering
adhesion
adhesive
ad hoc
ad infinitum
adipose
adiposity
adjacent
adjourn
adjournment
adjunct
adjust
adjustable
adjustment
adjuvant
Adler's theory
ad-lib
ad-libbed
ad-libbing
administer
administered

Aa

administering
administrate
administrated
administrating
administration
administrative
administrator
admirable
admirably
admiration
admire
admired
admiring
admissible
admissibly
admission
admit
admittance
admitted
admitting
admonish
adnexa
adnexal
adolescence
adolescent
adopt
adoption
adoptive
adrenal
adrenal cortex
adrenalectomize
adrenalectomy
adrenal hyperplasia
adrenaline
adrenal suppression
adrenarche
adrenergic
adrenoceptor
adrenocortical
adrenogenital
  syndrome
Adriamycin®

adrift
adroit
adsorb
adsorbent
adsorption
adsorptive
adult
adulterate
adulterated
adulterating
adulteration
advance
advanced
advancement
advancing
advantage
advantageous
advent
adventitia
adventitious
adventure
adventurous
adversaries
adversary
adverse
adverse reaction
adversities
adversity
advertise
advertised
advertisement
advertising
advice
advisability
advisable
advise
advised
advising
advisory
advocate
advocated
advocating

Aedes
Aedes aegypti
aegophony
aerate
aerated
aerating
aeration
aerial
aerobe
aerobic
aerobics
aerogenous
Aerolin®
aerophagia
aerophagy
aerosol
aetiological
aetiologically
aetiology
afebrile
affair
affect
affection
affectionate
affective
afferent
affiliate
affiliated
affiliating
affiliation
affinities
affinity
affirm
affirmation
affirmative
affix
afflict
affliction
affluent
afford
aflatoxin
afloat

afoot
aforesaid
afraid
Afrazine®
after-birth
aftercare
aftermath
afternoon
afterpains
aftertaste
afterthought
afterwards
again
against
agamma·
  globulinaemia
agamma·
  globulinaemic
aganglionosis
agar
Agarol®
age
aged
ageing
agencies
agency
agenda
agendas
agenesis
agent
agglutinate
agglutination
agglutinin
agglutinogen
aggravate
aggravated
aggravating
aggravation
aggression
aggressive
agile
agility

aging
agitate
agitated
agitating
agitation
agnosia
agonist
agonizing
agony
agoraphobia
agoraphobic
agranulocyte
agranulocytosis
agraphia
agraphic
agree
agreeable
agreeably
agreed
agreeing
agreement
agriculture
aground
ague
ahead
aid
AIDS
airborne
airily
airway
airways obstruction
airy
akathisia
akin
akinesia
akinesis
akinetic
Akineton®
alacrity
alanine
alarm
alarming

alarmist
albeit
Albers-Schönberg
  disease
albinism
albino
albinos
Albucid®
album
albumin
albuminuria
alchemy
alclometasone
  dipropionate
Alcoderm®
alcohol
alcohol-fast
alcoholic
Alcoholics
  Anonymous (AA)
alcoholism
alcoholuria
Alcopar®
alcuronium
Aldactide®
Aldactone®
aldehyde
aldolase
Aldomet®
aldosterone
aldosteronism
alert
aleukaemia
aleukaemic
alexia
alexic
alexitol
alfacalcidol
alfentanil
algae
Algicon®
alginate

Aa

Algipan®
alienate
alienated
alienating
alienation
align
alignment
alike
alimentary
alimentation
aliquot
alive
alkalaemia
alkalaemic
alkali
alkaline
alkalinity
alkalinization
alkalize
alkaloid
alkalosis
alkaptonuria
alkylating
alkylating agent
allantois
allegation
allege
alleged
allegiance
alleging
allele
allelomorph
allelomorphic
allelomorphism
allergen
allergenic
allergic
allergies
allergy
alleviate
alleviated
alleviating

alleviation
alliance
allocate
allocated
allocating
allocation
allograft
allopathy
allopurinol
allot
allotment
allotted
allotting
allow
allowable
allowance
alloy
all right
allude
alluded
alluding
allusion
Allyloestrenol
almasilate
Almevax®
almond oil
almoner
almost
aloe
alone
alopecia
Alopecia areata
Alopecia totalis
Alophen®
aloud
aloxiprin
alpha
alpha-adrenoceptor
alpha-adrenoceptor
  blocker
alphabet
alphabetical

alphabetically
alphachymotrypsin
Alphaderm®
alphafetoprotein
Alpha Keri®
alphanumeric
alphanumerical
alphatocopherol
alpha tocopheryl
  acetate
Alphosyl®
Alphosyl HC®
Alport's syndrome
alprazolam
alprostadil
already
Altacite Plus®
altar
alter
alteration
altercation
alter ego
alternans
alternate
alternated
alternately
alternating
alternation
alternative
alternatively
alternator
although
altitude
altogether
Alu-Cap®
Aludrox®
alum
aluminium
aluminium acetate
aluminium chloride
aluminium hydroxide
aluminosis

Alupent®
alveolar
alveoli
alveolitis
alveolus
alverine citrate
always
Alzheimer's disease
amalgam
amalgamate
amalgamated
amalgamating
amalgamation
amantadine
amass
amateur
amaurosis
amaurosis fugax
amaze
amazed
amazement
amazing
Ambaxin®
amber
ambidexterous
ambidextrous
ambiguities
ambiguity
ambiguous
ambition
ambitious
ambivalence
ambivalent
amblyopia
amblyopic
ambulance
ambulant
ambulatory
ambush
ambushes
Amelanotic melanoma
amelia

amelioration
amenable
amend
amendment
amenities
amenity
amenorrhoea
American
amethocaine
amiable
amiably
amicable
amicably
amid
amidst
amikacin
amiloride
amine
amino acid
aminoaciduria
aminobenzoate
aminobenzoic acid
aminocaproic
aminoglutethimide
aminoglycoside
aminopeptidase
aminophylline
amiodarone
amiss
amitosis
amitotic
amitriptyline
ammeter
ammonia
Ammonia
ammoniacal
ammonium
ammunition
amnesia
amnesic
amniocentesis
amnion

amnionitis
amniotic
amniotic cavity
amniotic fluid
amniotome
amniotomy
amodiaquine
amoeba
amoebae
amoebiasis
amoebic
amoebicidal
amoebicide
amoeboid
amoeboma
amok
among
amongst
amorphous
amount
Amoxil®
amoxycillin
amp
ampere
ampersand
amphetamine
amphotericin
ampicillin
Ampiclox®
ample
amplification
amplified
amplify
amplifying
amplitude
amply
ampoule
ampulla
ampullae
ampullar
ampullary
amputate

amputated
amputating
amputation
amputee
amsacrine
amuck
amygdala
Amygdaloid
amylase
amyl nitrite
amylobarbitone
amyloid
amyloidosis
amyotonia
amyotrophia
amyotrophy
Amytal®
anabolic
anabolism
anaemia
anaemic
anaerobe
anaerobic
anaesthesia
anaesthesiology
anaesthetic
anaesthetics
anaesthetist
anaesthetize
Anafranil®
anal
analeptic
analgesia
analgesic
analogies
analogous
analogue
analogy
analyse
analysed
analyser
analyses

analysing
analysis
analytic
analytically
anaphase
anaphylactic
anaphylactoid
anaphylactoid purpura
anaphylaxis
anaplasia
anaplastic
anarthria
anastomose
anastomoses
anastomosis
anastomotic
anatomical
anatomically
Anatomical snuffbox
anatomist
anatomy
ancestor
ancient
ancillary
ancrod
Ancylostoma
Ancylostoma
  duodenale®
ancylostomiasis
Androcur®
androgen
androgenic
androgenous
androstane
androstanediol
androstanediolone
androstanedione
androstene
androstenediol
androstenedione
androsterone
anecdote

anemometer
anemone
anencephalic
anencephalous
anencephaly
aneroid
aneurysm
aneurysmal
Anexate®
angelica
anger
angiitis
angina
anginal
angioblast
angioblastoma
angiogram
angiographic
angiographically
angiography
angioma
angiomatous
angioneurotic oedema
angiooedema
angiopathy
angioplasty
angiotensin
angiotensin-
  converting enzyme
  inhibitor
angle
angled
Angle of Louis
angling
angrily
angry
anguish
angular
angular stomatitis
anhidrosis
anhidrotic
anhydrase

Anhydrol Forte®
anhydrous
anicteric
aniline
animal
animate
animated
animating
animation
animosity
anion
anionic
aniseed
anisocytosis
ankle
ankylose
ankylosed
ankylosing spondylitis
ankylosis
Ankylostoma
annals
annex
annexe
annihilate
annihilated
annihilating
annihilation
anniversaries
anniversary
annotate
annotated
annotating
annotation
announce
announced
announcement
announcer
announcing
annoy
annoyance
annual
annually

annuals
annul
annular
annulare
annulate
annulled
annulling
annulment
annulus
anode
anogenital
anoint
anomalies
anomalopia
anomalous
anomaly
anomia
anonymity
anonymous
Anopheles
anoplasty
anorchia
anorchidism
anorchism
anorectal
anorectic
anorexia
anorexia nervosa
anorexic
anosmia
anosmic
another
anovular
anoxia
anoxic
Ansafone®
answer
answerable
Antabuse®
antacid
antagonism
antagonist

antagonistic
antagonize
antagonized
antagonizing
Antarctic
antazoline
antecedent
antecubital
antemortem
antenatal
antenatally
antenna
antennae
antennas
Antepar®
antepartum
anterior
anterolateral
anteroom
anteversion
antevert
anteverted
anthelmintic
Anthisan®
anthracosis
Anthranol®
anthraquinone
anthrax
anthropologist
anthropology
anthropometry
anthropomorphic
anti-androgen
anti-arrhythmic
antibacterial
antibiotic
antibodies
antibody
anticholinergic
anticholinesterase
anticipate
anticipated

anticipating
anticipation
anticlimax
anticlockwise
anticoagulant
anticonvulsant
anti-D
antidepressant
antidiabetic
antidiarrhoeal
antidiuretic
antidiuretic hormone
  (ADH)
antidote
antiemetic
antiepileptic
antifibrinolytic
antifungal
antigen
antigenic
antigenicity
antigiardial
antihepatitis B
antiherpes
antihistamine
antihypertensive
anti-infectious
anti-infective
anti-inflammatory
anti-Kell
antileprotic
antilymphocyte
antimalarial
antimetabolite
antimicrobial
antimigraine
antimony
antinuclear factor
anti-oestrogen
antiparasitic
antipathy
antiperspirant

antiplatelet
antiprotozoal
antipruritic
antipsychotic
antipyretic
antiquated
antique
antirabies
antirheumatic
antisepsis
antiseptic
antiserum
anti-smoking
antisocial
antispasmodic
antistatic
antistreptolysin
antitetanus
antitheses
antithesis
antithyroid
antitoxin
antituberculous
antitussive
antivaccinia
antivaricella
antivenom
antiviral
antizoster
Antraderm®
antrectomy
antroscopy
antrostomy
antrotome
antrotomy
antrum
Anturan®
Anugesic-HC®
anuria
anuric
anus
Anusol®

Anusol-HC®
anxieties
anxiety
anxiolytic
anxious
anybody
anyhow
anyone
anything
anywhere
aorta
aortic
aortitis
aortogram
aortography
aortopulmonary
apart
apathetic
apathy
aperient
Apert's disease or
  syndrome
aperture
apex
apexes
Apgar
aphagia
aphagic
aphakia
aphakic
aphasia
aphasic
aphonia
aphonic
aphrodisiac
aphthous
aphthous ulcer
apical
apices
apiece
Apisate®
aplasia

aplastic
apnoea
apnoeic
apocrine
apoenzyme
apologetic
apologetically
apologies
apologize
apologized
apologizing
apology
apomorphine
aponeuroses
aponeurosis
aponeurotic
apophyseal
apophysis
apoplectic
apoplexy
apothecaries
apothecary
appal
appalled
appalling
apparatus
apparel
apparent
apparently
appeal
appear
appearance
appease
appeased
appeasing
append
appendage
appendectomy
appendicectomy
appendices
appendicitis
appendicular

appendix
appendixes
appetite
appetizing
applaud
appliance
applicable
applicant
application
applicator
applied
apply
applying
appoint
appointment
apportion
apposite
apposition
appraisal
appraise
appraised
appraising
appreciable
appreciably
appreciate
appreciated
appreciating
appreciation
apprehend
apprehension
apprehensive
approach
approachable
approaches
approbation
appropriate
appropriated
appropriating
approval
approve
approved
approving

approximate
approximately
approximation
apractic
apraxia
apraxic
Apresoline®
April
Aprinox®
apropos of
aptitude
apyrexia
apyrexial
aqua
aquaria
aquarium
aquariums
aquatic
aqueduct
aqueous
arabinose
arachidonic acid
arachis oil
arachnodactyly
arachnoid
arachnoidal
arachnoiditis
arbitrarily
arbitrary
arbitrate
arbitrated
arbitrating
arbitration
arbitrator
arborization
arbovirus
arc
arcade
arch
archaeologist
archaeology
archaic

arches
archetype
architect
architectural
architecturally
architecture
archives
Arctic
arcuate
arcus senilis
ardent
arduous
arduousness
area
areas
areatus
arena
aren't
areola
areolar
argentaffin
argentaffinoma
arginine
argipressin
argon
arguable
arguably
argue
argued
arguing
argument
argumentative
Argyll Robertson pupil
argyria
arid
arise
arisen
arising
arithmetic
armaments
armies
armoured

armoury
army
Arnold-Chiari
  malformation
aroma
aromatic
arose
around
arouse
aroused
arousing
arrange
arranged
arrangement
arranging
arrectores pilorum
arrector pili
arrest
arrhenoblastoma
arrhythmia
arrival
arrive
arrived
arriving
arrogant
arrow
arsenic
arsenical
Artane®
artefact
arterectomy
arterial
arteries
arteriogram
arteriographic
arteriographically
arteriography
arteriolar
arteriole
arteriopuncture
arteriosclerosis
arteriosclerotic

arteriospasm
arteriostenosis
arteriovenous
arteritis
artery
arthralgia
arthralgic
arthritic
arthritis
arthrodesis
arthrogram
arthrographic
arthrographically
arthrography
arthrogryposis
arthropathy
arthroplastic
arthroplasty
arthropod
arthroscope
arthroscopic
arthroscopy
arthrosis
arthrotomy
article
articular
articulate
articulated
articulating
articulation
artifact
artificial
artificiality
artificially
artistry
artless
arytenoid
asbestos
asbestosis
ascariasis
ascaricide
ascarides

ascaris
Ascaris lumbricoides
ascend
ascendancy
ascendant
ascendency
ascendent
ascent
ascertain
Aschoff's nodules
ascites
ascitic
ascorbic acid
ascribe
ascribed
ascribing
asepsis
aseptic
Aserbine®
asexual
ashamed
ashen
aside
Asilone®
askance
askew
asleep
asparaginase
aspartase
aspect
Aspellin®
aspergillosis
Aspergillus
asphalt
asphyxia
asphyxiate
asphyxiated
asphyxiating
asphyxiation
aspirate
aspiration
aspirator

aspirin
assailant
assassin
assassinate
assassinated
assassinating
assassination
assault
assay
assemble
assembled
assemblies
assembling
assembly
assent
assert
assertion
assertive
assertiveness
assess
assessment
assessor
asset
assiduous
assign
assignation
assignment
assimilate
assimilated
assimilating
assimilation
assist
assistance
assistant
assisted
associate
associated
associating
association
assorted
assortment
assuage

assuaged
assuaging
assume
assumed
assuming
assumption
assurance
assure
assured
assuring
astemizole
astereognosis
asterisk
asthenia
asthenic
asthma
asthmatic
asthmatically
astigmatic
astigmatism
astonish
astound
astringency
astringent
astrocyte
astrocytoma
astronomical
astronomically
astronomy
Astrup
astute
asunder
asylum
asymmetry
asymptomatic
asystole
Atarax®
atavism
ataxia
ataxic
ate
atelectasis

atelectatic
Atenolol
atheist
atherogenesis
atherogenic
atheroma
atheromatous
atherosclerosis
atherosclerotic
athetoid
athetosis
athetotic
athlete
athlete's foot
athletics
Ativan®
atlantal
atlanto-axial
atlanto-occipital
atlas
Atmocol®
atmosphere
atmospheric
atmospherically
atmospherics
atom
atomic
atomizer
atonia
atonic
atonicity
atopic
atracurium
atresia
atresic
atria
atrial
atrial fibrillation
atrial flutter
atrial septal defect
atrioventricular
atrium

atrocious
atrocities
atrocity
Atromid-S®
atrophic
atrophied
atrophy
atropine
Atrovent®
attach
attaché-case
attachment
attack
attacker
attain
attainable
attainment
attempt
attend
attendance
attendant
attention
attentive
attenuate
attenuated
attenuation
attic
attitude
attract
attraction
attractive
attributable
attribute
attributed
attributing
attrition
atypical
audacity
audibility
audible
audibly
Audicort

audience
audiogram
audiological
audiologically
audiology
audiometer
audiometric
audiometrist
audiometry
audio-typist
audio-visual
audit
auditor
auditoria
auditorium
auditoriums
auditory
Auerbach
au fait
augment
Augmentin
August
aura
aural
auranofin
Aureocort®
Aureomycin®
auricle
auricular
auriculotemporal
auriscope
aurothiomalate
auscultate
auscultation
auscultatory
auspices
auspicious
austere
austerity
Austin Flint murmur
Australian
Austrian

authentic
authenticate
authenticated
authenticating
authenticity
author
authoritarian
authoritative
authorities
authority
authorization
authorize
authorized
authorizing
autism
autistic
auto-agglutination
auto-analyser
auto-antibody
auto-antigen
autoclave
auto-immune
auto-immunization
autolysis
automata
automatic
automatically
automation
automatism
automaton
automatons
autonomic
autonomous
autonomy
autopsies
autopsy
autosensitization
autosomal
autosome
autosuggestion
autotransfusion
autumn

auxiliaries
auxiliary
avail
availability
available
avascular
avascularization
Aveeno®
avenue
average
averaged
averaging
averse
aversion
aversion therapy
avert
avian
avid
avitaminosis
Avloclor®
avoid
avoidable
avoidably
avoidance
Avomine®
avow
avowal
avulsion
await
awake
awaken
award
aware
awareness
awesome
awful
awfully
awfulness
awkward
awkwardly
awkwardness
awoke

awry
axe
axed
axes
axial
axilla
axillary
axing
axis
axis-cylinder
axle
axon
axonal
Ayre's spatula
azapropazone
azatadine
azathioprine
azidothymidine
azlocillin
azoospermia
AZT
aztreonam
azygos

Bb

babies
Babinski's reflex
baboon
baby
babyhood
babysat
babysit
babysitter
babysitting
bacampicillin
bachelor
bachelorhood

Bb

bacillary dysentery
Bacille-Calmette-
  Guérin
bacilli
bacillus
Bacillus anthracis
backer
background
backing
backward
backwards
baclofen
bacteraemia
bacteraemic
bacteria
bacterial
bactericidal
bactericide
bacteriological
bacteriologically
bacteriologist
bacteriology
bacteriolysin
bacteriophage
bacteriostatic
bacterium
bacteriuria
Bacteroides
Bactigras®
Bactrim®
bad
bade
baffle
baffled
baffling
baggage
bake
baked
Baker's cyst
baking
BAL
balance

balanced
balancing
balanitis
balconies
balcony
bald
baldness
bale
balk
Balkan beam
Balkan frame
balked
balking
ballast
ballet
ballistic
balloon
ballooning
ballot
ballottable
ballottement
balm
Balneum®
balsam
balsa wood
ban
banal
banalities
banality
banana
bandage
bandaged
bandaging
bandied
bandy
bandying
bandy(-legged)
banish
banister
bank-note
bankrupt
bankruptcy

banned
banner
banning
banns
banquet
bar
barb
barbaric
barbarically
barbed
barber
barbiturate
bare
barely
bargain
barium
baroceptor
barometer
baroreceptors
barracuda
Barr body
barred
barrel
barren
barrenness
barricade
barricaded
barricading
barrier
barring
barter
bartholinitis
Bartholin's glands
basal
basal ganglia
base
based
bases
basic
basically
basilar
basilic

basin
basing
basis
basket
basophil
basophilia
basophilic
bass
basses
bat
batch
batches
bated
bathe
bathed
bathing
batted
battered baby
  syndrome
batteries
battering
battery
batting
baulk
baulked
baulking
beach
beaches
beading
beaker
beam
bear
bearable
beard
bearded
bearer
bearing
bearing-down
beast
beat
beaten
beauties

beautiful
beautifully
beauty
became
because
beckon
beclomethasone
  dipropionate
Becodisks®
become
becoming
Beconase®
Becotide®
bed
bedbug
bedded
bedding
bedpan
bedridden
bed-sit
bed-sitter
bedsore
been
beeswax
beeturia
befit
befitted
befitting
before
beforehand
befriend
beg
began
begged
begging
begin
beginning
begrudge
begrudged
begrudging
beguile
beguiled

beguiling
begun
behalf
behave
behaved
behaving
behaviour
behavioural
behaviourist
Behçet's disease or
  syndrome
behind
beholden
beige
being
bejel
belated
belch
belching
beleaguer
beleaguered
Belgian
belie
belied
belief
believe
believed
believing
belittle
belittled
belittling
belladonna
'belle indifférence'
bellies
belligerent
bellows
Bell's palsy
belly
belong
belongings
beloved
below

belying
Bence-Jones protein
bench
benches
bend
bending
bendrofluazide
bends
beneath
Benedict's solution
benefactor
beneficially
beneficiaries
beneficiary
benefit
benefited
benefiting
Benemid®
Benerva®
benign
Bennett's fracture
Benoral®
benorylate
benoxinate
Benoxyl®
benperidol
benserazide
bent
bentonite
Benylin®
benzalkonium chloride
benzathine penicillin
benzene
benzhexol
benzoate
benzocaine
benzodiazepine
benzoic acid
benzoin tincture
benzoyl peroxide
benztropine
benzydamine

benzyl benzoate
benzyl penicillin
Beogex®
bephenium
bereaved
bereavement
bereft
bergamot oil
beri-beri
Berotec®
berries
berry
berserk
berth
Bertiella
berylliosis
beset
besetting
beside
besides
Besnier's prurigo
best
bestow
beta
beta-adrenoceptor
beta-blocker
Betadine®
betahistine
beta-lactamase
Betaloc®
betamethasone
betamethasone
    dipropionate
betamethasone
    valerate
betanin
betaxolol
betel
bethanechol
bethanidine
Betnesol®
Betnesol-N®

Betnovate®
Betnovate-C®
Betnovate-N®
Betnovate-RD®
betray
betrayal
better
bettered
bettering
betting
between
bevel
bevelled
bevelling
beverage
beware
Bextasol®
beyond
bezafibrate
bias
biased
biasing
biassed
biassing
bibliographer
bibliographies
bibliography
bicarbonate
bicentenary
biceps
bicipital
biconcave
biconvex
bicornuate
bicuspid
bicycle
bid
bidding
bidet
biennial
biennially
Bier's method

bifid
bifocal
bifurcate
bifurcation
bigemina
bigeminal
bigeminous
bigeminy
bigger
biggest
bigoted
bigotry
biguanide
bike
bilateral
bilaterally
bile
bilge
Bilharzia
bilharziasis
biliary
biliary-tract
bilingual
bilious
biliousness
bilirubin
bilirubinaemia
biliverdin
billion
Billroth's operation
bilobate
bilobular
biluria
bimanual
binary
binaural
bind
binder
binding
Binet's test
binocular
binovular

BiNovum®
bio-assay
biochemical
biochemistry
biodegradable
bioengineering
biofeedback
Biogastrone®
biographical
biographies
biography
biological
biologically
biologist
biology
biopsy
biorhythm
biosynthesis
biotechnically
biotechnology
biotin
biparietal
biperiden
biphasic
bipolar
birch
birches
birth
birthday
birthmark
bisacodyl
biscuit
bisect
bisection
bisexual
bisexuality
bismuth
bisoprolol
bit
bitch
bitches
bite

bitten
bitter
bitters
bivalent
bivalve
bi-weekly
bizarre
black
blacken
blackhead
blackout
blackwater fever
bladder
blade
Blalock's operation
blame
blamed
blameless
blaming
blanch
bland
blank
blanket
blasphemous
blastocoele
blastocyte
blastoma
blastomere
Blastomyces
blastomycosis
blastula
blatant
bleach
bleaches
bleak
bleary
bleb
bled
bleed
bleeder
bleeding
'bleeding time'

Bb

bleep
blemish
blemishes
blend
blender
bleomycin
blepharitis
blepharoconjunctivitis
blepharoplasty
blepharospasm
blew
blight
blighted ovum
blind
blindfold
blind loop syndrome
blindness
blink
blister
bloated
blob
block
blockade
blockaded
blockading
blond
blonde
blood
blood-brain barrier
blood-letting
bloodshed
bloodshot
bloody
blot
blotch
blotches
blotchy
blotted
blotting
blow
blowing
blown

blubber
blue
blueprint
bluff
blunt
blur
blurred
blurring
blush
blushes
BM stix
BM-Test Glycemie 1-44
boa constrictor
board
boarder
boast
bodies
bodily
bodily harm
body
bodyguard
body-surface
body-weight
bogus
boil
boiler
bold
bolt
bolus
Bolvidon®
bomb
bombard
bombardment
bombshell
bona fide
bona fides
bond
bone
bone-chips
bone-marrow
bonfire
Bonjela®

bonus
bonuses
bony
bookkeeping
booklet
boon
boost
booster
boot
booth
borax
borborygmi
border
Bordetella
Bordetella pertussis
Bordet-Gengou
bore
bored
boredom
boric acid
boring
born
borne
Bornholm disease
borough
Borrelia
Borrelia vincenti
borrow
bosom
boss
bosses
botanical
botanically
botanist
botany
botch
both
bother
bottle
bottled
bottleneck
bottling

bottom
botulinum
botulinus
botulism
bought
bougie
bougienage
bounce
bounced
bouncing
bound
boundaries
boundary
bounded
bounding
bouquet
bout
bouton
boutonnière
bovine
bow
bowed
bowel
bowels
Bowen's disease
bowing
bowl
box
boxes
boycott
boyhood
boyish
Boyle's anaesthetic
  machine
brace
braced
braces
brachial
brachialis
brachiocephalic
brachioradialis
bracing

bracket
bracketed
bracketing
Bradilan®
bradycardia
bradykinesis
bradykinetic
bradykinin
bradyrhythmia
braid
braille
brain
brainstorm
brainwave
brainy
braise
braised
braising
brake
braked
braking
bran
branch
branches
branchial
brand
brandish
brand-new
Brandt Andrews
  technique
brassière
brave
braved
bravery
braving
breach
breaches
bread
breadth
break
breakable
breakage

breakfast
breaking
breast
breast-feeding
breath
breathalyser
breathe
breathed
breathing
breathless
bred
breech
breeches
breed
breeding
breeze
breezy
bretylium
Brevinor®
brevity
brew
Bricanyl®
brick
bridge
bridged
bridging
brief
brigade
bright
Bright's disease
brilliance
brilliant
brilliant
brimful
brine
bring
bringing
brink
brisk
bristly
Britain
British

Briton
brittle
broach
broad
broadcast
broadcasting
broaden
Broca's area
brochure
Brodie's abscess
broke
broken
Brolene®
bromal
bromazepam
bromelain
bromide
bromocriptine
bromosulphthalein
brompheniramine
Brompton cocktail
bronchi
bronchial
bronchiectasis
bronchiectatic
bronchiolar
bronchiole
bronchiolitis
bronchitic
bronchitis
bronchoconstrictor
bronchodilator
bronchogenic
bronchogram
bronchography
broncholith
bronchopneumonia
bronchopneumonic
bronchopulmonary
bronchoscope
bronchoscopic
bronchoscopically

bronchoscopy
bronchospasm
bronchus
bronze
bronzed
brood
brook
brother
brotherhood
brother-in-law
brotherly
brothers-in-law
brought
brow
brown
Brown-Séquard
  disease
brucella
Brucella abortus
Brucella melitensis
brucellosis
Brufen®
bruise
bruised
bruising
bruit
brunette
brunt
brush
brushes
brusque
brutal
brutality
brutally
brute
bubble
bubbled
bubbling
bubo
bubonic
buccal
buccinator

bucket
buckle
buckled
buckling
buckshot
Budd-Chiari disease
budesonide
budget
budgetary
budgeted
budgeting
Buerger's disease
buffer
buffet
buffeted
buffeting
build
builder
building
built
built-up
bulb
bulbar
bulbospongiosus
bulbourethral
bulbous
bulge
bulged
bulging
bulimia
bulimia nervosa
bulk
bulk-forming
bulky
bulla
bullae
bullet
bulletin
bullied
bullies
bullous
bully

bullying
bumble-bee
bumetanide
bump
bunch
bunches
bundle
bundled
bundling
bunion
bunk
bunk-bed
Bunsen burner
buoy
buoyancy
buoyant
buphthalmos
bupivacaine
buprenorphine
bur
burden
bureau
bureaucracies
bureaucracy
bureaucratic
bureaus
bureaux
burgh
burglar
burial
buried
Burinex®
Burinex K®
Burkitt's lymphoma
burly
burn
burned
burner
burning
burnout syndrome
burnt
burr

bursa
bursae
bursitis
burst
bursting
bury
burying
Buscopan®
buserelin
bush
bushes
bushy
busier
busiest
busily
business
businesses
businessman
buspirone
bust
busulphan
busy
Butacote®
Butazolidin®
Butazone®
butobarbitone
butriptyline
butt
butter
butterflies
butterfly
buttock
button
buttonhole
butyraldehyde
butyrate
butyrophenone
butyrophenones
buy
buyer
buying
buzzer

bye-law
by-election
bygone
by-law
bypass
by-product
byssinosis
bystander
byte

Cc

cab
cabin
cabinet
cable
cache
cachectic
cachexia
cadaver
cadaveric
cadaverous
cadence
cadet
cadmium
caecal
caecostomy
caecotomy
caecum
caeruloplasmin
caesarean section
caesium
café
Cafergot®
cafeteria
cafeterias
caffeine
cage

caged
cagey
caging
cagy
cake
caked
caking
Calaband®
Caladryl®
calamine
calamities
calamitous
calamity
calcaneal
calcanean
calcaneum
calcareous
calceal
Calichew®
calciferol
calcification
calcitonin
calcitriol
calcium
calcium alginate
calcium-channel
Calcium-Sandoz®
calculate
calculated
calculating
calculation
calculator
calculi
calculosis
calculous
calculus
Caldwell-Luc
  operation
calendar
calf
calibrate
calibrated

calibrating
calibre
caliper
calipers
callipers
callisthenics
callithenics
callosity
callosum
callous
callus
calluses
calm
calmness
Calmurid®
Calmurid HC®
calor
caloric test
calorie
calorific
calorimeter
calorimetry
Calpol®
calves
calyceal
calyces
calyx
Camcolit®
camera
camomile
camouflage
camouflaged
camouflaging
campaign
Campbell De Morgan
camphor
camphorated
campus
campuses
Campylobacter
Campylobacter
  enteritis

canal
canalicular
canaliculi
canaliculization
canaliculus
canalization
canal of Schlemm
cancel
cancelled
cancelling
cancellous
cancer
cancerophobia
cancerophobic
cancerous
cancrum oris
candid
Candida
Candida albicans
candidacy
candidate
candidiasis
candidosis
candies
candle
candour
candy
cane
caned
Canesten®
Canesten-HC®
canine
caning
canister
canker
cankerous
cannabis
canned
cannibal
cannibalism
canning
cannon

cannonball
cannot
cannula
cannulae
cannulate
cannulation
canoe
canoes
canon
canopies
canopy
can't
canteen
canthal
canthi
canthus
canton
canvas
canvases
canvass
canvassed
canvassing
cap
capabilities
capability
capable
capacious
capacities
capacity
cape
Capgras' syndrome
Capillaria
capillariasis
capillaries
capillary
capital
capitalism
capitalist
capitalistic
capitalization
capitalize
capitalized

capitalizing
capitate
capitulate
capitulated
capitulating
capitulation
capitulum
Caplans' syndrome
Capoten®
Capozide®
capped
capping
capreomycin
capsize
capsized
capsizing
capsular
capsule
capsulectomy
capsulitis
capsulotomy
captain
captaincies
captaincy
caption
captivate
captivated
captivating
captive
captivity
captopril
captor
capture
captured
capturing
caput succedaneum
Carace®
carafe
caramel
carat
caravan
caraway

carbachol
carbamazepine
carbaryl
carbenicillin
carbenoxolone
carbidopa
carbimazole
carbocisteine
Carbo-Dome®
carbohydrate
carbolic
carbon
carbonate
carbonic anhydrase
carbon monoxide
carbonmonoxyhaemo·
   globin
carboplatin
Carborundum
carboxyhaemoglobin
carboxyhaemoglobin·
   aemia
carboxyhaemoglobin·
   uria
carboxymethyl·
   cellulose
carbuncle
carburetter
carburettor
carcase
carcass
carcinogen
carcinogenesis
carcinogenic
carcinogenicity
carcinoid
carcinoma
carcinomata
carcinomatosis
carcinomatous
card
cardboard

cardia
cardiac
cardiac arrest
cardigan
cardinal
cardiogenic
cardiogram
cardiograph
cardiography
cardio-inhibitory
cardiolipin
cardiologist
cardiology
cardiomegaly
cardiomyopathic
cardiomyopathy
cardiopulmonary
cardiorespiratory
cardiospasm
cardiothoracic
cardiotocograph
cardiotocography
cardiotomy
cardiotoxic
cardiovascular
cardioversion
carditis
care
cared
career
careful
carefully
carefulness
careless
caress
caresses
caretaker
careworn
carfecillin
cargo
cargoes
caricature

caricaturist
caries
carina
carinal
caring
cariogenic
carious
carisoprodol
carmellose
carmustine
carnage
carnal knowledge
carnation
carneous mole
carnival
carnivore
carnivorous
carotenaemia
carotenes
carotenoids
carotid
carpal
carpal tunnel
carpal tunnel
  syndrome
carpenter
carpentry
carpet
carpeted
carpeting
carpometacarpal
carpopedal
carpus
carriage
carried
carrier
carry
carrying
carte blanche
cartel
carteolol
cartilage

cartilaginous
cartography
carton
cartoon
cartridge
cartwheel
caruncle
caruncula
caruncular
carve
carved
carving
cascara
case
caseate
caseation
cased
casein
caseinogen
casement
caseous
caseous degeneration
cash
cashier
casing
casket
Casoni test
casserole
cassette
cassock
cast
castaway
caste
Castellani's paint
caster
caster sugar
casting
castle
cast-off
castor
castor-oil
castrate

castrated
castrating
castration
casual
casually
casualties
casualty
catabolic
catabolism
catabolite
catacomb
catagen
catalase
catalogue
catalogued
cataloguing
catalysis
catalyst
catalytic
cataplectic
cataplexy
cataract
catarrh
catarrhal
catastrophe
catastrophic
catastrophically
catatonia
catatonic
catch
catching
catchment
catchy
catecholamine
categorical
categorically
categories
category
cater
catered
caterer
catering

catgut
catharsis
cathartic
catheter
catheterization
catheterize
cathode
cathode ray tube
cation
cattle
cauda
cauda equina
caudal
caudate
caught
caul
cauldron
cauliflower
causalgia
cause
caused
causing
caustic
caustically
cauterization
cauterize
cauterized
cauterizing
cautery
caution
cautionary
cautious
cavalcade
cavalry
cave
Caved-S®
cavern
cavernous
cavitation
cavities
cavity
cavort

cayenne
Ceanel®
cease
ceased
ceaseless
ceasing
cedar
cede
ceded
ceding
Ceefax®
cefaclor
cefadroxil
cefotaxime
cefoxitin
cefsulodin
ceftazidime
ceftizoxime
cefuroxime
ceiling
celebrate
celebrated
celebrating
celebration
celebrities
celebrity
Celevac®
celibate
cell
cell mediated
  immunity
cellophane
cellular
cellulicidal
cellulitis
celluloid
cellulose
cellulose wadding
Celsius
cement
censor
censure

censured
censuring
census
censuses
cent
centenarian
centenaries
centenary
centigrade
centigram
centigramme
centilitre
centimetre
central
centralization
centralize
centralized
centralizing
centrally
centre
centrifugal
centrifuge
centriole
centripetal
centromere
centuries
century
Centyl®
Centyl K®
cephalexin
cephalic
cephalin
cephalhaematoma
cephalosporin
cephalothin
cephalotome
cephamandole
cephamycin
cephazolin
cephradine
Ceporex®
ceramic

ceratonia
cercocystis
cereal
cerebellar
cerebellopontine
cerebellum
cerebral
cerebration
cerebropontine
cerebrospinal
cerebrovascular
cerebrum
ceremonies
ceremony
cereous
certain
certainly
certainties
certainty
certificate
certified
certify
certifying
ceruloplasmin
cerumen
ceruminous
Cerumol®
cervical
cervicitis
cervix
cessation
cestode
Cetavlon®
Cetavlon PC®
Cetiprin®
cetomacrogol
cetrimide
cetylpyridinium
C-Film®
chafe
chafed
chafing

Chagas' disease
chagoma
chain
chair
chairman
chalazion
chalk
chalky
challenge
challenged
challenging
chalone
chamber
champagne
champion
championship
chance
chanced
chancellor
chancing
chancre
chancroid
change
changeable
changed
changing
channel
channelled
channelling
chaos
chaotic
chaotically
chapped
chapter
char
character
characteristic
characteristically
characterize
characterized
characterizing
charcoal

Charcot-Marie-Tooth
Charcot's disease
  or joint
charge
chargeable
charged
charging
charitable
charitably
charities
charity
charm
charming
Charnley's arthrodesis
charred
charring
chart
charter
charwoman
chary
chase
chased
chasing
chasm
chassis
chaste
chastity
chat
chatted
chatting
chauffeur
cheap
cheapen
cheat
check
checked
checkmate
check-out
cheek
cheekily
cheeky
cheerful

cheerfully
cheese
cheetah
chef
cheilitis
cheiloplasty
cheilosis
cheiropompholyx
cheiropractic
cheiropractor
cheiropraxis
chelate
chelating agent
chelation
chemical
chemically
chemist
chemistry
chemoprophylactic
chemoprophylaxis
chemoreceptor
chemosensitive
chemosis
chemosuppression
chemotactic
chemotaxis
chemotherapeutic
chemotherapy
chemotic
chemotransmitter
chenodeoxycholic
  acid
cheque
chequered
cherish
chest
chew
Cheyne-Stokes
  respiration
chiasma
chicken
chicken-pox

chicory
chid
chide
chided
chiding
chief
chiefly
chilblain
child
childhood
childish
childlike
children
child-resistant
chili
chilies
chill
chilli
chillies
chilly
chimaera
chime
chimed
chimera
chiming
chimney
china
Chinese
chink
chip
chipped
chipping
Chiron®
Chironair®
chiropodist
chiropody
chiropractic
chiropractor
chirp
chisel
chiselled
chiselling

chit
chive
Chlamydia
Chlamydia
  trachomatis
chloasma
chloral hydrate
chlorambucil
chloramphenicol
chlordiazepoxide
chlorhexidine
chloride
chlorinate
chlorinated
chlorinating
chlorination
chlorine
chlormethiazole
chlormezanone
chloroform
chloroma
Chloromycetin®
chlorophyll
chloroquine
chlorothiazide
chlorothymol
chloroxylenol
chlorpheniramine
chlorpromazine
chlorpropamide
chlortetracycline
chlorthalidone
choana
choanae
choanal
chock-full
chocolate
choice
choke
choked
choking
cholagogue

cholangiogram
cholangiographic
cholangiography
cholangiohepatitis
cholangitis
cholecalciferol
cholecystagogue
cholecystectomy
cholecystitis
cholecystoduoden·
  ostomy
cholecystogram
cholecystography
cholecystokinin
cholecystostomy
choledochoduodenal
choledocholithiasis
choledocholithotomy
choledochostomy
choledochotomy
cholelithiasis
cholera
choleric
cholestasis
cholestatic
cholesteatoma
cholesterol
cholestyramine
choline
choline magnesium
  trisalicylate
cholinergic
choline salicylate
cholinesterase
choline theophyllinate
choluric
chondral
chondritis
chondroblast
chondrocostal
chondrocyte
chondrodynia

chondrolysis
chondroma
chondromalacia
chondromatosis
chondromatous
chondrosarcoma
chondrosarcomata
chondrosarcomatous
chondrosternal
choose
choosing
chop
chopped
chopping
chord
chordee
chorditis
chordotomy
chore
chorea
choreiform
choreo-athetoid
choreo-athetosis
choriocarcinoma
chorion
chorionic
chorionic villus
chorioretinitis
choroid
choroidal
choroiditis
choroidoretinal
choroidoretinitis
chorus
choruses
chose
chosen
Christian
Christmas
Christmas disease
chromaffin
chromaffinoma

chromatic
chromatid
chromatin
chromatogram
chromatography
chrome
chromic
chromium
chromocentre
chromophil
chromophobe
chromosomal
chromosome
chronic
chronically
chronicity
chronicle
chronological
chronologically
chronometer
chrysalis
chubby
chunk
church
churches
chute
Chvostek's sign
chyle
chylothorax
chymase
chyme
chymosin
chymotrypsin
chymotrypsinogen
Cicatrin®
cicatrix
cicatrization
cicatrize
ciclacillin
cigar
cigarette
cilastatin

cilia
cilial
ciliary
ciliated
cimetidine
cinder
cineangiocardio·
   graphy
cineangiography
cingulum
cinnamon
cinnarizine
cinoxacin
ciprofloxacin
circa
circadian rhythm
circinate
circle
circled
circle of Willis
circling
circuit
circuitous
circular
circulate
circulated
circulating
circulation
circulatory
circumcision
circumference
circumflex
circumoral
circumorally
circumscribed
circumspect
circumstances
circumstantial
circumstantiality
circumvallate
circumvent
cirrhosis

cirrhotic
cirsoid
cisplatin
cisterna
cisternal
citation
cite
cited
cities
citing
citizen
citrate
citric acid
citrus fruit
city
civic
civil
civilian
civilities
civility
civilization
civilize
civilized
civilizing
civilly
clad
claim
claimant
clammy
clamour
clandestine
clap
clapped
clapping
clarified
clarify
clarifying
clarity
clash
clashes
class
classes

classic
classical
classically
classification
classified
classify
classifying
claudication
clause
claustrophobia
claustrophobic
clavicle
clavicular
clavulanic
clavulanic acid
claw-foot
claw-hand
clean
cleaner
cleanliness
cleanness
cleanse
cleansed
cleansing
clear
clearance
clearly
clearness
cleft
cleft palate
clemastine
clench
clerical
clerk
clever
cleverness
cliché
click
client
clientele
Clifton Assessment
climacteric

climate
climatic
climax
climaxes
climb
clindamycin
cling
clinging
clinic
clinical
clinically
clink
Clinoril®
clioquinol
clip
clipped
clipping
clique
clitoral
clitoris
cloaca
cloacal
cloak
clobazam
clobetasol propionate
clobetasone butyrate
clock
clockwise
clockwork
clofazimine
clofibrate
clog
clogged
clogging
cloistered
Clomid®
clomiphene
clomipramine
clomocycline
clonazepam
clone
clonic

clonidine
clonus
clopamide
clopenthixol
Clopixol®
clorazepate
close
closed
closed-angle
  glaucoma
closely
closeness
closet
close-up
closing
Clostridium
Clostridium botulinum
Clostridium difficile
Clostridium tetani
Clostridium welchii
closure
clot
cloth
clothe
clothed
clothes
clothing
clotrimazole
clotted
clotting
cloud
cloudy
clove
clover
clown
cloxacillin
club
clubbed
clubbing
club-foot
clue
clump

clumping
clumsily
clumsiness
clumsy
clung
cluster
clutch
clutches
coach
coaches
coagulase
coagulate
coagulated
coagulating
coagulation
coagulum
coalesce
coalesced
coalescence
coalescent
coalescing
coalfield
coalition
coal tar
coarctation
coarse
coarsen
coast
coastal
coat
coax
cobalt
cobbler
Co-Betaloc®
cobra
cobweb
cocaine
coccal
cocci
coccidioidomycosis
coccus
coccydynia

coccygeal
coccygectomy
coccygeus
coccyx
cochineal
cochlea
cochlear
cock
cockatoo
cockerel
cocker spaniel
cockily
cockle
cockpit
cockroach
cockroaches
cocksure
cocktail
cocky
cocoa
co-codamol
co-codaprin
coconut
cocoon
co-danthramer
co-danthrusate
code
codeine
co-dergocrine
  mesylate
Codis®
co-driver
co-dydramol
coeducation
coefficient
coeliac
co-enzyme
coerce
coerced
coercing
coercion
coeur en sabot

co-exist
co-existence
coffee
coffee ground vomit
cogent
Cogentin®
cognac
cognition
cognizance
cohabitation
coherent
cohesion
cohesive
coiffure
coil
coin
coinage
coincide
coincided
coincidence
coincidental
coinciding
coital
coitus
coitus interruptus
coke
colander
colchicine
cold
coldness
cold sore
colectomy
cole-slaw
Colestid®
colestipol
colic
colicky
Colifoam®
coliform
colistin
colitis
collaborate

collaborated
collaborating
collaboration
collagen
collagenase
collagenosis
collagenous
collapse
collapsed
collapsible
collapsing
collar
collar-bone
collate
collated
collateral
collating
colleague
collect
collection
collective
collector
college
Colles' fracture
colliculus
collide
collided
colliding
collision
collodion
colloid
colloidal
colloquial
colloquialism
colloquially
collusion
coloboma
colobomata
colocolic
Colofac®
colon
colonel

colonial
colonic
colonies
colonist
colonize
colonoscope
colonoscopy
colony
colorectal
colorimeter
colorimetric
colorimetry
colossal
colostomy
Colostomy®
colostrum
colour
colourful
colourfully
Colpermin®
colpoperineorrhaphy
colpoplasty
colporrhaphy
colposcope
colposcopically
colposcopy
column
columnar
coma
comatose
combat
combatant
combated
combating
combination
combine
combined
combined oral
   contraceptive
combining
combustible
combustion

come
comedian
comedies
comedo
comedone
comedones
comedy
Comfeel®
comfort
comfortable
comfortably
comic
comical
comically
coming
comma
command
commander
commemorate
commemorated
commemorating
commemoration
commence
commenced
commencement
commencing
commend
commendable
commendation
commensal
commensurate
comment
commentaries
commentary
commentator
commerce
commercial
commercially
comminuted
commiserate
commiserated
commiserating

commission
commissionaire
commissioner
commissure
commissurotomy
commit
commitment
committal
committed
committee
committing
commodities
commodity
common
commoner
commonplace
Commonwealth
commotion
communal
communicable
communicans
communicate
communicated
communicating
communication
communicative
communion
communities
community
commute
commuted
commuter
commuting
compact
companies
companion
company
comparable
comparably
comparative
compare
compared

comparing
comparison
compartment
compass
compasses
compassionate
compatibility
compatible
compatibly
compel
compelled
compelling
compensate
compensated
compensating
compensation
compete
competed
competence
competent
competing
competition
competitive
competitor
compilation
compile
compiled
compiling
complacent
complain
complement
complementary
complement fixation
  test
complete
completed
completing
completion
complex
complexes
complexion
complexities

complexity
compliance
compliant
complicate
complicated
complicating
complication
complied
compliment
complimentary
Comploment
  Continus®
comply
complying
component
compose
composed
composing
composite
composition
compos mentis
composure
compound
comprehend
comprehensible
comprehension
comprehensive
compress
compression
compressor
comprise
comprised
comprising
compromise
compromised
compromising
compulsion
compulsive
compulsorily
compulsory
compute
computed

computed axial
  tomography
computer
computerized axial
  tomography
computing
comrade
concave
conceal
concede
conceded
conceding
conceit
conceited
conceivable
conceivably
conceive
conceived
conceiving
concentrate
concentrated
concentrating
concentration
concentric
concept
conception
conceptus
concern
concerted
concession
conciliate
conciliated
conciliating
conciliation
concise
conclude
concluded
concluding
conclusion
conclusive
concoct
concoction

concomitant
concord
Concordin®
concrete
concretion
conctractile
concur
concurred
concurrent
concurring
concussion
condemn
condemnation
condensation
condense
condensed
condensing
condescend
condescending
condescension
condiment
condition
conditional
conditionally
conditioned
conditioning
condolences
condom
condone
condoned
condoning
conducive
conduct
conductance
conductibility
conduction
conductivity
conductor
conductress
conductresses
conduit
condylar

condyle
condyloma
condylomatous
coney
confabulation
confection
confectioner
confectionery
confederate
confederation
confer
conference
conferred
conferring
confess
confession
confide
confided
confidence
confident
confidential
confidentially
confiding
configuration
confine
confined
confinement
confines
confining
confirm
confirmation
confiscate
confiscated
confiscating
confiscation
conflict
confluence
confluent
conform
conforming
conformity
confound

confront
confrontation
confuse
confused
confusing
confusion
congeal
congealed
congealing
congener
congenial
congenially
congenital
conger-eel
congested
congestion
congestive
conglomerate
conglomeration
congratulate
congratulated
congratulating
congratulations
congregate
congregated
congregating
congregation
congress
congresses
congruent
conical
conization
conjugal
conjugate
conjugated
conjunction
conjunctiva
conjunctival
conjunctivitis
connect
connection
connective

connoisseur
connotation
Conn's syndrome
Conotrane®
Conova 30®
conquer
conqueror
conquest
consanguineous
consanguinity
conscience
conscientious
conscientiousness
conscious
consciousness
conscript
conscription
consecutive
consensual
consensus
consent
consequence
consequent
consequently
conservation
conservationist
conservative
conservatories
conservatory
conserve
conserved
conserving
consider
considerable
considerably
considerate
consideration
consign
consignment
consist
consistency
consistent

consolation
console
consoled
consolidate
consolidated
consolidating
consolidation
consoling
consonant
consort
consortium
conspicuous
conspiracies
conspiracy
conspire
conspired
conspiring
constable
constancy
constant
constipate
constipation
constituencies
constituency
constituent
constitute
constituted
constituting
constraint
constrict
constrictor
construct
construction
constructive
consult
consultant
consultation
consume
consumed
consumer
consuming
consumption

consumptive
contact
contagion
contagious
contain
container
contaminant
contaminate
contaminated
contaminating
contamination
contemplate
contemplated
contemplating
contemplative
contemporaneous
contemporary
contempt
contemptible
contemptibly
contemptuous
contend
content
contented
contention
context
contiguity
contiguous
continence
continent
contingencies
contingency
contingent
continual
continually
continuance
continuation
continue
continued
continuing
continuity
continuous

continuous
  ambulatory
  peritoneal
  dialysis
  (CAPD)
contort
contortion
contour
contraception
contraceptive
contract
contractile
contractility
contraction
contracture
contradict
contradictory
contraindication
contralateral
contralaterally
contraption
contrary
contrast
contrastimulant
contrastimulus
contrast media
contravene
contravened
contravening
contrecoup
contribute
contributed
contributing
contribution
contributor
control
controlled
controller
controlling
controversial
controversially
controversies

controversy
Controvlar®
contuse
contusion
conus
convalesce
convalesced
convalescence
convalescent
convalescing
convection
convene
convened
convener
convenience
convenient
convening
convention
conversant
conversation
conversational
conversationally
conversion
convert
converter
convertible
convex
convexity
convey
conveyance
conveyed
conveying
conveyor belt
convict
conviction
convince
convinced
convincing
convoluted
convolution
convoy
convulsant

convulse
convulsed
convulsing
convulsion
convulsive
cony
cooker
cookery
cooking
cool
Cooley's anaemia
coolly
coolness
Coombs' test
co-operate
co-operated
co-operating
co-operation
co-operative
co-opt
co-opted
co-opting
co-ordinate
co-ordinated
co-ordinating
co-ordination
cope
coped
copied
copies
coping
copious
copper
Coppertone Super·
   shade 15®
Coppertone Ultra·
   shade 23®
coprolalia
coproporphyria
coproporphyrin
coproporphyrinuria
co-proxamol

copulation
copy
copying
copyright
coraco-acromial
coracobrachialis
coracoclavicular
coracoid
coral
cord
Cordarone X®
cordectomy
cordial
cordiality
cordially
Cordilox®
cordon
cordon bleu
cordotomy
corduroy
core
cored
co-respondent
Corgard®
Corgaretic®
coring
cork
corkscrew
Corlan®
corm
cornea
corneal
corneas
corner
corner-stone
cornflour
cornu
corollaries
corollary
coronal
coronaries
coronary

corona virus
coroner
corpora
corporal
Corpora lutea
corporate
corporation
corps
corpse
corpses
corpulence
corpulent
cor pulmonale
corpus
corpus callosum
corpuscle
corpuscular
Corpus luteum
Corpus spongiosum
correct
correction
corrective
correlated
correlation
correspond
correspondence
correspondent
corridor
corroborate
corroborated
corroborating
corroboration
corrode
corroded
corroding
corrosion
corrosive
corrugated
corrupt
corruptible
corruption
corset

Corsodyl®
cortex
cortical
corticate
cortices
corticopontine
corticospinal
corticosteroid
corticothalamic
corticotrophic
corticotrophin
cortisol
cortisone
cortisone acetate
Corwin®
Corynebacterium
Corynebacterium
  diphtheriae
coryza
cosily
cosmetic
cosmetology
cosmopolitan
cost
costal
costed
costing
costive
costly
costochondral
costochondritis
costoclavicular
costophrenic
costume
cosy
Cotazym®
co-trimoxazole
cottage
cotton
cotton-wool
cotyledon
couch

couches
cough
could
coumarin
council
councillor
counsel
counselled
counselling
counsellor
count
countenance
countenanced
countenancing
counter
counteract
counter-extension
counterfeit
counterfoil
counter-irritant
counter-irritation
countermand
counterpart
countershock
countersign
countertraction
counties
countless
countries
country
countryside
county
coup
couple
coupled
coupling
coupon
courage
courageous
courier
course
court

courteous
courtesy
courtyard
Courvoisier's law
cousin
couvade
Couvelaire uterus
covenant
cover
coverage
covering
Covermark®
covert
coward
cowardice
cowardly
cowboy
cowl
Cowper's glands
cowpox
cox
coxa
coxalgia
Coxa plana
Coxa valga
Coxa vara
Coxiella
Coxiella burnetti
coxodynia
Coxsackie
Coxsackie virus
coxswain
crab
crab louse
crack
cracker
crackle
crackled
crackling
cradle
cradle cap
cradled

cradling
craft
craftily
craftsman
crafty
cram
crammed
cramming
cramp
cramped
cranial
craniectomy
craniopharyngioma
cranioplasty
craniostenosis
craniostosis
craniosynostosis
craniotabes
craniotabetic
craniotomy
cranium
crannies
cranny
crape
crash
crashes
crass
crate
crated
crater
crating
crave
craved
craving
crawl
crayon
craze
crazily
crazy
c-reactive protein
creak
cream

crease
creased
creasing
create
created
creatinase
creatine
creatine kinase
creating
creatinine
creatinuria
creation
creative
creator
creature
crèche
credentials
credibility
credible
credibly
credit
creditable
credited
crediting
creditor
credulity
credulous
creed
creep
creeping
cremaster
cremasteric
cremate
cremated
cremating
cremation
crematorium
crenate
crenated
crenation
Creon®
creosote

crepe
crepitation
crepitus
crept
crescent
crestfallen
cretin
cretinism
Creutzfeldt-Jakob
  disease
crevasse
crevice
crew
cribriform
crick
crico-arytenoid
cricohyoid
cricoid
'cri du chat'
  syndrome
cried
cries
Crigler-Najjar
  syndrome
crime
criminal
criminal abortion
criminally
crimson
cripple
crippled
crippling
crisantaspase
crises
crisis
crisp
crispy
criss-cross
crista
criteria
criterion
critic

critical
critically
criticism
criticize
criticized
criticizing
croak
crockery
crocodile
crocus
crocuses
Crohn's disease
cromoglycate
Crooke's hyaline
  cells
crop
cropped
cropping
Crosby capsule
cross
crosses
cross-examine
cross-examined
cross-examining
cross-infection
crossing
cross-matching
crossroads
cross-section
crotamiton
crouch
croup
croupy
crowbar
crowd
crowded
crown
crucial
crucially
cruciate
crucified
crucifix

crucifixes
crucifixion
crucify
crucifying
crude
crudity
cruel
cruelly
cruelty
cruise
cruised
cruiser
cruising
crumb
crumble
crumbled
crumbling
crumple
crumpled
crumpling
crunch
crura
crural
crus
crusade
crush
crust
crustacean
crusty
crutch
crutches
crux
cry
crying
cryoanalgesia
cryogenic
cryoglobulin
cryoprecipitate
cryoprobe
cryosurgery
cryotherapy
cryptic

cryptically
cryptococcosis
Cryptococcus
cryptogenic
cryptomenorrhoea
cryptorchid
cryptorchism
crystal
crystallin
crystalline
crystallization
crystallize
crystallized
crystallizing
crystalluria
crystal violet
Crystapen®
cubic
cubicle
cubital
cubitus
cuboid
cuboidal
cucumber
cue
cuff
cufflinks
cuirass
cuisine
cul-de-sac
culdoscope
culdoscopy
culinary
culminate
culminated
culminating
culmination
culpable
culprit
cultivate
cultivated
cultivating

cultivation
culture
cumulative
cuneate
cuneiform
cunnilinction
cunning
cup
cupboard
cupful
Cuplex®
cupped
cupping
curable
curare
curarize
curb
curdle
curdled
curdling
cure
cured
curettage
curette
curetting
curie
curing
curiosities
curiosity
curious
Curling's ulcer
currencies
currency
current
curricula
curricula vitae
curriculum
curriculums
curriculum vitae
curse
cursed
cursing

cursor
cursorily
cursory
curtail
curvature
curve
curved
curving
Cusco's speculum
cushingoid
Cushing's disease
  or syndrome
cushion
cusp
custodian
custody
custom
customarily
customary
customer
cut
cutaneous
cuticle
cuticular
cutting
cyanide
cyanocobalamin
cyanosed
cyanosis
cyanotic
cybernetics
cyclamate
cyclandelate
cycle
cycled
cyclical
Cyclimorph®
cycling
cyclist
cyclitis
cyclizine
cyclobarbitone

cyclofenil
cycloid
cyclone
cyclopenthiazide
cyclopentolate
cyclophosphamide
cycloplegia
cycloplegic
Cyclo-Progynova®
cyclopropane
cycloserine
Cyclospasmol®
cyclosporin
cyclothyme
cyclothymia
cyclothymic
cyclotomy
cyclotron
cyesis
Cyklokapron®
cylinder
cylindrical
cylindrically
cylindroma
cymbal
Cymevene®
cynic
cynical
cynically
cynicism
cyproheptadine
cyproterone acetate
cyst
cystadenoma
cystectomy
cysteine
cystic
cysticercosis
cysticercus
cystic fibrosis
cystiform

cystine
cystinosis
cystinuria
cystitis
cystitome
cystocele
cystogram
cystolithiasis
cystometrogram
cystometry
cystopexy
cystoscope
cystoscopic
cystoscopically
cystoscopy
cystostomy
cystotomy
Cytamen®
cytarabine
cytogenetics
cytological
cytology
cytolysis
cytolytic
cytomegalovirus
cytomegaly
cytopathic
cytopathology
cytoplasm
cytoplasmic
cytoscopically
cytosine
cytotoxic
cytotoxin
cytotrophoblast
Czech

Dd

dab
dabbed
dabbing
dacarbazine
dachshund
dacryocystectomy
dacryocystitis
dacryocystography
dacryocystorhin‐
  ostomy
dactinomycin
daddies
daddy
daffodil
dagger
dahlia
dailies
daily
daintily
daintiness
dainty
dairies
dairy
dais
daises
daisies
daisy
daisy-wheel
Dakin's solution
Daktacort®
Daktarin®
Dalacin C®
dale
Dalmane®
damage
damaged
damaging
dame

damn
damnation
damp
dampen
damper
dampness
danazol
dance
danced
dancer
dancing
dandelion
dandruff
Daneral-SA®
danger
dangerous
dangle
dangled
dangling
Danish
Danol®
Danol-1/2®
danthron
Dantrium®
dantrolene
Daonil®
dapsone
Daraprim®
dare
dared
Darier's disease
daring
darken
darkness
dartboard
dartos muscle
Darwinism
dash
dashes
dashing
data
database

date
dated
dating
datum
daughter
daughter-in-law
daughters-in-law
daunt
dauntless
dawn
daydream
daze
dazed
dazing
dazzle
dazzled
dazzling
deactivation
dead
deaden
deadline
deadliness
deadly
deaf
deafen
deafened
deafening
deaf-mute
deaf-mutism
deafness
deal
dealcoholization
dealer
dealing
dealt
dearness
dearth
death
deathly
debar
debarred
debarring

debase
debased
debasement
debasing
debatable
debate
debated
debating
debilitate
debilitated
debilitating
debility
debit
débridement
debris
Debrisan®
debrisoquine
debt
debtor
debug
début
debutante
decade
decadence
decadent
Deca-Durabolin®
decalcification
decalcify
decanoate
decapitate
decapitated
decapitating
decarboxylase
decay
decayed
decaying
decease
deceased
deceit
deceitful
deceitfully
deceive

deceived
deceiving
decelerate
decelerated
decelerating
December
decency
decent
deception
deceptive
decerebrate
decibel
decide
decided
decidedly
deciding
decidua
decidual
deciduous
decilitre
decimal
decimate
decimated
decimating
decimolar
decipher
decision
decisive
declaration
declare
declared
declaring
Declinax®
decline
declined
declining
decode
decoded
decoding
decolorize
decompensation
decompose

decomposed
decomposing
decomposition
decompression
deconditioning
decongestant
decongestion
décor
decorate
decorated
decorating
decoration
decorative
decorator
decortication
decrease
decreased
decreasing
decree
decreed
decreeing
decrepit
decrepitude
decrudescence
decubital
decubitus
decussation
dedicate
dedicated
dedicating
dedication
deduce
deduced
deducing
deduct
deduction
deed
deepen
deer
deface
defaced
defacing

defaecate
defaecation
defamation
defamatory
defame
defamed
defaming
default
defaulter
defeat
defect
defection
defective
defectiveness
defence
defenceless
defend
defendant
defensible
defensive
defer
deference
deferens
deferent
deferential
deferentially
deferred
deferring
defiance
defiant
defibrillate
defibrillation
defibrillator
defibrinated
deficiencies
deficiency
deficient
deficit
defied
define
defined
defining

definite
definitely
definition
definitive
deflate
deflated
deflating
deflect
deflection
deform
deformation
deformed
deformities
deformity
defraud
defrost
defunct
defusion
defy
defying
degeneracy
degenerate
degeneration
degenerative
degloving
deglutition
degradation
degree
degustation
dehiscence
dehumanization
dehydrate
dehydrated
dehydrating
dehydration
dehydrocholic acid
dehydrogenase
deign
déjà vu
dejected
dejection
delay

delegate
delegated
delegating
delegation
delete
deleted
deleting
deletion
Delfen®
deliberate
deliberated
deliberately
deliberating
deliberation
delicacies
delicacy
delicate
delicious
delight
delinquent
deliquescence
deliquescent
delirious
delirium
deliver
deliverance
deliveries
delivery
delouse
Deltacortril®
deltoid
delude
deluded
deluding
deluge
deluged
deluging
delusion
delusional
demand
demarcation
demarkation

demeanour
demecarium bromide
demeclocycline
dement
demented
dementia
dementia praecox
demineralization
demise
democracies
democracy
democrat
democratic
democratically
demography
demolish
demolition
demonstrable
demonstrably
demonstrate
demonstrated
demonstrating
demonstration
demonstrative
demonstrator
demoralize
demoralized
demoralizing
demote
demoted
demoting
demulcent
demyelinate
demyelination
demyelinization
denaturation
denatured
dendrite
dendritic
denervate
denervation
dengue

denial
denied
denier
Denis Browne's splint
De-Nol®
denomination
denominational
denominator
denote
denoted
denoting
denounce
denounced
denouncing
dense
densities
density
dental
dentate
dentifrice
dentine
dentist
dentistry
dentition
denture
denucleated
denudation
denude
denunciation
deny
denying
deodorant
deodorize
deossification
deoxidation
deoxidize
deoxygenation
deoxyribonucleic acid
  (DNA)
depart
department
departure

depend
dependable
dependant
dependence
dependent
depersonalization
depict
depigmentation
depilate
depilation
depilatory
Depixol®
deplete
depleted
depleting
depletion
deplorable
deplorably
deplore
deplored
deploring
Depocillin®
depolarizing
depolarization
depolarize
Depo-Medrone®
Depo-Provera®
depopulated
deport
deportation
depose
deposed
deposing
deposit
depositories
depository
Depostat®
depot
depravation
depreciate
depreciated
depreciating

depreciation
depress
depression
deprivation
deprive
deprived
depriving
deprogram
depth
deputation
deputies
deputize
deputized
deputizing
deputy
Dequadin®
dequalinium
deranged
derangement
Derbac-C®
derealization
derelict
dereliction
deride
derided
deriding
derision
derisive
derive
derived
deriving
dermabrasion
Dermacolor®
dermal
dermatitis
dermatitis artefacta
dermatitis
  herpetiformis
dermatitis
  medicamentosa
dermatofibroma
dermatographia

dermatographism
dermatological
dermatologically
dermatologist
dermatology
dermatome
dermatomyositis
dermatophyte
dermatoses
dermatosis
dermis
dermographia
dermographic
dermoid
Dermovate®
derogatorily
derogatory
descend
descendant
descendent
descending
descent
describe
described
describing
description
descriptive
desensitization
desensitize
desert
deserter
desertion
deserve
deserved
deserving
desferrioxamine
desiccant
desiccate
desiccated
desiccating
desiccation
design

designate
designated
designating
designation
desipramine
desirable
desirably
desire
desired
desiring
desist
desloughing
desmopressin
desogestrel
desolate
desolation
desonide
desoxymethasone
despair
despatch
despatches
desperate
desperately
desperation
despicable
despicably
despise
despised
despising
despite
despondency
despondent
desquamate
desquamation
dessertspoonful
destination
destined
destiny
destitute
destroy
destructible
destruction

destructive
desultorily
desultory
detach
detachable
detached retina
detachment
detail
detain
Deteclo®
detect
detection
detective
detector
detention
deter
detergent
deteriorate
deteriorated
deteriorating
deterioration
determination
determine
determined
determining
deterred
deterrent
deterring
detest
detestable
detestably
detour
detoxicant
detoxicate
detoxication
detoxify
detract
detraction
detriment
detrimental
detrition
detritus

detrusor
Dettol®
devaluation
devascularization
devastate
devastated
devastating
devastation
develop
developed
developer
developing
development
deviance
deviate
deviated
deviating
deviation
device
devilish
devious
devise
devised
devising
devoid
devote
devoted
devoting
devotion
devour
dexamethasone
dexamphetamine
Dexedrine®
dexterity
dexterous
dextoposition
dextran
dextranomer
dextrocardia
dextromethorphan
dextromoramide
dextroposition

dextropropoxyphene
dextrose
dextrothyroxine
dextrous
DF 118
diabetes
diabetes insipidus
diabetes mellitus
diabetic
diabetogenic
Diabinese®
diagnose
diagnosed
diagnoses
diagnosing
diagnosis
diagnostic
diagnostician
diagonal
diagonally
diagram
diagrammatic
dial
dialect
dialled
dialling
dialogue
dialysate
dialyse
dialyser
dialysis
diameter
diamorphine
Diamox®
Diane®
Dianette®
diaphragm
diaphragmatic
diaphyseal
diaphyses
diaphysis
diaries

diarrhoea
diarrhoeal
diarthrosis
diary
diastase
diastasis
diastole
diastolic
diathermy
diathesis
diazepam
diazoxide
dice
dichloralphenazone
dichlorphenamide
dichotomy
diclofenac
dicobalt edetate
Diconal®
dicrotic
Dictaphone®
dictate
dictated
dictating
dictation
diction
dictionaries
dictionary
dicyclomine
  hydrochloride
die
died
diencephalon
dienoestrol
diesel
diet
dietary
dietetic
dietetics
diethylcarbamazine
diethyl ether
diethylpropion

dietitian
differ
difference
different
differential
differentiate
differentiated
differentiating
differentiation
difficult
difficulties
difficulty
Difflam®
diffraction
diffusate
diffuse
diffusibility
diffusible
diffusion
Diflucan®
diflucortolone
  valerate
diflunisal
dig
digastric
digest
digestibility
digestible
digestion
digestive
digging
digit
digital
digitalis
digitalism
digitalization
digitate
digitoxin
dignified
digoxin
digress
digression

dihydrochloride
dihydrocodeine
dihydroergotamine
dihydrotachysterol
dihydroxycholecal·
  ciferol
dike
dilatation
dilate
dilated
dilating
dilation
dilator
dilemma
diligence
diligent
diloxanide furoate
diltiazem
diluent
dilute
diluted
diluting
dilution
dim
dimenhydrinate
dimension
dimensional
dimercaprol
dimethicone
dimethindene
dimethyl sulphoxide
diminish
diminution
diminutive
dimmed
dimming
dimorphic
dimorphism
dimorphous
Dimotane®
dimple
Dindevan®

dine
dined
dining
dinner
dinoprost
dinoprostone
Dioctyl®
diode
Diogenes syndrome
dioptre
Dioralyte®
dip
diphenoxylate
diphenylbutyl·
  piperidine
diphenylpyraline
diphosphanate
diphtheria
diphtheritic
diphtheroid
diphthong
Diphyllobothrium
dipipanone
dipivefrine
diplegia
diplegic
diplococcal
diplococcus
diploic
diploid
diploma
diplomacy
diplomat
diplopia
dipole
dipped
dipping
Diprobase®
Diprosone®
dipsomania
dipsomaniac
Diptera

dipyridamole
dire
direct
direction
director
directories
directory
dirt
dirtied
dirtily
dirtiness
dirty
dirtying
disabilities
disability
disable
disabled
disablement
Disablement
  Resettlement Officer
  (DRO)
disabling
disaccharidase
disaccharide
disadvantage
disadvantageous
disaffected
disaggregation
disagree
disagreeable
disagreeably
disagreed
disagreeing
disagreement
Disalcid®
disallow
disappear
disappearance
disappeared
disappearing
disappoint
disappointed

Dd

disappointment
disapproval
disapprove
disapproved
disapproving
disarrange
disarranged
disarranging
disarray
disarticulation
disassociation
disaster
disastrous
disband
disbelief
disbelieve
disbelieved
disbelieving
disc
discard
discectomy
discern
discernible
discernibly
discerning
discharge
discharged
discharging
disciform
disciple
disciplinarian
disciplinary
discipline
discitis
disclaim
disclaimer
disclose
disclosed
disclosing
disclosing tablet
disclosure
discoid

discolour
discolouration
discoloured
discolouring
discomfort
disconcert
disconnect
disconnection
disconsolate
discontent
discontinue
discontinued
discontinuing
discord
discordant
discount
discourage
discouraged
discouraging
discourteous
discover
discoveries
discovery
discredit
discreet
discrepancies
discrepancy
discrete
discretion
discriminate
discriminated
discriminating
discrimination
discuss
discussion
disdain
disease
diseased
disembodied
disengage
disengaged
disengagement

disengaging
disentangle
disentangled
disentangling
disequilibrium
disfavour
disfigure
disfigured
disfiguring
disgrace
disgraced
disgraceful
disgracefully
disgracing
disgruntled
disguise
disguised
disguising
disgust
disgusted
dish
dishes
dishevelled
dishonest
dishonesty
dishonour
dishonourable
dishonourably
disillate
disillusion
disillusioned
disillusioning
disimpaction
disinclined
disinfect
disinfectant
disinfection
disinfestation
disinhibited
disinhibition
disintegrate
disintegrated

disintegrating
disintegration
disinterested
Disipal®
disjointed
disjunction
disjunctive
disk
diskette
dislike
disliked
disliking
dislocate
dislocated
dislocating
dislocation
dismantle
dismantled
dismantling
dismay
dismember
dismembered
dismembering
dismemberment
dismiss
dismissal
disobedience
disobedient
disobey
disobeyed
disobeying
disobliging
disodium etidronate
disopyramide
disorder
disorderliness
disorderly
disorientation
disown
disparage
disparaged
disparagement

disparaging
disparities
disparity
dispatch
dispatches
dispel
dispelled
dispelling
dispensable
dispensaries
dispensary
dispensation
dispense
dispensed
dispenser
dispensing
dispersal
disperse
dispersed
dispersible
dispersing
dispersion
displace
displaced
displacement
displacing
display
displease
displeased
displeasing
displeasure
disposable
disposal
dispose
disposed
disposing
disposition
dispossess
Disprol®
disproportion
disproportionate
disprove

dispute
disputed
disputing
disqualification
disqualified
disqualify
disqualifying
disquieting
disregard
disrepair
disreputable
disreputably
disrespect
disrespectful
disrupt
disruption
disruptive
dissatisfaction
dissatisfied
dissatisfy
dissatisfying
dissect
dissection
dissector
disseminated
dissemination
dissension
dissent
dissenter
dissertation
disservice
dissimilar
dissimilarities
dissimilarity
dissimilation
dissimulate
dissimulated
dissimulating
dissipate
dissipated
dissipating
dissipation

dissociate
dissociated
dissociating
dissociation
dissolute
dissolution
dissolve
dissolved
dissolving
dissonance
dissuade
dissuaded
dissuading
Distaclor®
distal
Distalgesic®
distally
distance
distant
distaste
distemper
distend
distension
distigmine
distil
distillate
distillation
distilled
distilleries
distillery
distilling
distinct
distinction
distinctive
distinguish
distort
distortion
distract
distractibility
distraction
distraught
distress

distribute
distributed
distributing
distribution
district
distrust
disturb
disturbance
disulfiram
disuse
disused
ditch
ditches
dithranol
Dithrocream®
ditto
Diumide-K ®
diuresis
diuretic
diurnal
divan
divarication
diverge
diverged
divergence
divergent
diverging
diverse
diversification
diversified
diversify
diversifying
diversion
diversity
divert
diverticula
diverticular
diverticulitis
diverticulosis
diverticulum
divide
divided

dividend
dividing
divinities
divinity
divisible
division
divisional
divorce
divorced
divorcee
divorcing
divulge
divulged
divulging
Dixarit®
dizziness
dizzy
dobutamine
docile
docket
doctor
doctrine
document
documentaries
documentary
docusate sodium
dodge
dodged
dodging
doer
does
dogma
dogmatic
dogmatically
doing
doldrums
dole
doleful
dolefully
dolefulness
dollar
dollies

dolly
Dolobid®
dolor
Doloxene®
dolphin
domain
dome
Dome-Acne®
domestic
domestically
domesticated
domesticity
domicile
dominance
dominant
dominate
dominated
dominating
domination
domineering
dominion
domino
dominoes
domperidone
donate
donated
donating
donation
donator
done
donkey
donor
Donovan's body
don't
dopa-decarboxylase
dopamine
dopaminergic
dope
doped
doping
Doppler ultrasound
  technique

Doptone®
Dor®
dormancy
dormant
dormice
dormitories
dormitory
dormouse
dorsal
dorsalis
dorsiflexion
dorsolumbar
dorsosacral
dorsum
dosage
dose
dosed
dosemeter
dosing
dossier
dotage
dothiepin
dotted
double
doubled
doublet
doubling
doubly
doubt
doubted
doubtful
doubting
doubtless
douche
dough
doughnut
dovetail
downfall
Down's syndrome
downstairs
downtime
downtrodden

downwards
doxapram
doxepin
doxorubicin
doxycycline
dozen
dracontiasis
dracunculosis
Dracunculus
Dracunculus
  medinensis
draft
drag
dragged
dragging
dragonflies
dragonfly
drain
drainage
drama
Dramamine®
dramas
dramatic
dramatically
dramatist
drank
Drapolene®
drastic
drastically
draught
draughty
draw
drawer
drawing
drawn
drawsheet
dread
dreadful
dreadfully
dream
dreamed
dreamily

dreaming
dreamt
dreamy
dregs
drench
dressing
drew
Driclor®
dried
drill
drily
drink
drinking
drip
dripped
dripping
drip-set
drive
driven
driver
driving
drop
droperidol
droplet
dropped
dropper
dropping
droppings
dropsy
Drosophila
drostanolone
drought
drove
drown
drowsily
drowsy
drug
drugged
drugging
druggist
drum
drummed

drumming
drunk
drunkard
drunken
drunkenness
dry
dry-clean
dry-cleaned
dry-cleaning
drying
dryly
dual
dub
dubbed
dubbing
Dubin-Johnson
  syndrome
dubious
Duchenne muscular
  dystrophy
duct
ductus arteriosus
due
duel
duellist
dues
duet
duffel coat
dug
duke
Dulcolax®
dull
dully
duly
dumb
dumbfound
dumbness
dummies
dummy
dumping
'dumping syndrome'
dunce

dune
dungarees
dungeon
duodenal
duodenitis
duodenojejunal
duodenoscope
duodenoscopic
duodenoscopy
duodenostomy
duodenum
Duofilm®
Duovent®
dupe
duped
Duphalac®
Duphaston®
duping
duplicate
duplicated
duplicating
duplication
duplicity
Dupuytren's
  contracture
dura
durable
durably
Durabolin®
Duracreme®
Duragel®
dural
dura mater
duration
duress
during
Duromine®
Durules®
duster
Dutch
dutiable
duties

dutiful
dutifully
duty
Duvadilan®
dwarf
dwarfism
dwarfs
dwarves
dwell
dwelled
dwelling
dwelt
dwindle
dwindled
dwindling
Dyazide®
dydrogesterone
dye
dyed
dyeing
dyestuff
dying
dyke
dynamic
dynamite
dynamo
dynamometer
dynamos
dynastic
dynasties
dynasty
dysaesthesia
dysarthria
dysarthric
dyscalculia
dyschezia
dyschondroplasia
dyscrasia
dysenteric
dysentery
dysfunction
dysfunctional

dysgenesis
dysgerminoma
dyskaryosis
dyskinesia
dyskinetic
dyslalia
dyslalic
dyslexia
dyslexic
dysmaturity
dysmelia
dysmenorrhoea
dysmnesia
dysmnesic
dysmorphia
dysmorphism
dysmorphogenic
dysmorphosis
dysostosis
dyspareunia
dyspepsia
dyspeptic
dysphagia
dysphagic
dysphasia
dysphonia
dysphoria
dysplasia
dysplastic
dyspnoea
dyspnoeic
dyspraxia
dyspraxic
dysrhythmia
dysrhythmic
dystocia
dystonia
dystonic
dystrophia myotonica
dystrophic
dystrophy
dysuria

Ee

E45®
eager
earache
eardrops
eardrum
earl
earlier
earliest
earliness
early
earmark
earn
earnest
earnings
earth
earthenware
earthly
earthquake
earwig
ease
eased
easel
easier
easiest
easily
easing
east
Easter
easterly
eastern
eastward
eastwards
easy
eat
eatable
eaten
eating
eaves

eavesdrop
eavesdropped
eavesdropping
ebony
Ebstein's anomaly
ebullient
eccentric
eccentricities
eccentricity
ecchondroma
ecchondromata
ecchymoses
ecchymosis
Echinococcus
echo
echocardiography
echoencephalography
echoes
echolalia
echolalic
echopraxia
echovirus
eclampsia
eclamptic
eclectic
eclecticism
eclipse
eclipsed
eclipsing
ecological
ecologically
ecologist
ecology
Econacort®
econazole
economic
economical
economically
economics
economies
economist
economize

economized
economizing
economy
ecopthiopate iodide
Ecostatin®
ecstasies
ecstasy
ectoderm
ectodermal
ectomorphy
ectoparasite
ectopia
ectopic
ectoplasm
ectropion
Eczederm®
eczema
eczematization
eczematous
eczema vaccinatum
eddies
eddy
Edecrin®
edentulous
edge
edged
edgeways
edgily
edging
edgy
edible
edict
edifice
Edinger-Westphal
  nucleus
edit
edition
editor
editorial
editorially
edrophonium
educate

educated
educating
education
educational
educationally
educationally
  subnormal (ESN)
Edward syndrome
eeriness
Efcortelan®
effect
effective
effectively
effectiveness
effector
effectual
effectually
efferent
effervesce
effervesced
effervescence
effervescent
effervescing
efficacious
efficacy
efficiency
efficient
efflorescence
efflorescent
effluent
effluvium
effort
effrontery
effusion
ego
egocentric
egoism
egoist
egoistic
egoistically
egotism
egotist

egotistic
egotistically
Ehlers-Danlos
  syndrome
Ehrlich's reagent
eiderdown
eider duck
eight
eighteen
eighteenth
eighth
eightieth
eighty
Einthoven's formula
either
ejaculate
ejaculated
ejaculating
ejaculation
ejaculatory
eject
ejection
ejector
eked out
eke out
eking out
elaborate
elaborated
elaborating
elapse
elapsed
elapsing
elastase
elastic
elasticated
elasticity
elastin
Elastoplast®
elbow
elder
eldest
elect

election
elective
electocution
electorate
Electra complex
electric
electrical
electrically
electrician
electricity
electrified
electrify
electrifying
electrocardiogram
  (ECG)
electrocardiograph
electrocardiographic
electrocardiograph·
  ically
electrocardiography
electrocautery
electroconvulsive
electroconvulsive
  therapy (ECT)
electrocute
electrocuted
electrocuting
electrocution
electrode
electroencephalo·
  gram (EEG)
electroencephalo·
  graph
electroencephalo·
  graphic
electroencephalo·
  graphically
electroencephalo·
  graphy
electrolysis
electrolyte
electrolytic

electromagnetism
electron
electronic
electronically
electronics
electronystagmogram
electronystagmo·
  graphy
electrophoresis
electrophoretic
elegance
elegant
element
Elemental®
elementary
elephant
elephantiasis
elevate
elevated
elevating
elevation
elevator
eleven
elevenses
eleventh
elicit
eligibility
eligible
eliminate
eliminated
eliminating
elimination
ELISA
élite
elixir
ellipse
ellipses
elliptical
elliptically
elliptocyte
elliptocytosis
elocution

elongation
eloquent
elsewhere
Eltroxin®
elucidate
elucidated
elucidating
Eludril®
elusive
emaciate
emaciated
emaciation
emanate
emanated
emanating
emanation
emancipate
emancipated
emancipating
emancipation
emasculation
embalm
embankment
embargo
embargoes
embark
embarkation
embarrass
embarrassed
embarrassing
embarrassment
embassies
embassy
ember
embezzle
embezzled
embezzling
emblem
embodied
embodiment
embody
embodying

embolectomy
emboli
embolic
embolism
embologenic
embolus
emboss
embrace
embraced
embracing
embrocation
embroider
embroidery
embroil
embryo
embryological
embryologically
embryology
embryonic
embryos
emerald
emerge
emerged
emergence
emergencies
emergency
emergent
emerging
emery
emesis
emetic
emetine
Emetrol®
emigrant
emigrate
emigration
eminence
eminent
eminently
emission
emit
emitted

emitting
emmetropia
emmetropic
emollient
emolument
emotion
emotional
emotionally
empathic
empathize
empathy
emphasis
emphasize
emphasized
emphasizing
emphatic
emphatically
emphysema
emphysematous
empire
empirical
empirically
empiricism
employ
employee
employer
employment
emptied
empties
emptiness
empty
emptying
empyema
emulate
emulated
emulating
Emulsiderm®
emulsification
emulsifier
emulsify
emulsifying
emulsion

enable
enabled
enabling
enact
enalapril
enamel
enamelled
enamelling
Enanthate
encampment
encaphalin
encapsulation
encephalin
encephalitis
encephalitis lethargica
encephalocele
encephalogram
encephalography
encephalomyelitis
encephalon
encephalopathic
encephalopathy
enchondroma
enchondromata
enclave
enclose
enclosed
enclosing
enclosure
encompass
encopresis
encopretic
encounter
encounter group
encourage
encouraged
encouraging
encroach
encumbrance
encyclopaedia
encyclopaedic
encyclopedia

encyclopedic
encyst
endanger
endarterectomy
endarteritis
endeavour
En-De-Kay ®
endemic
endemiology
endocardial
endocarditis
endocardium
endocervical
endocervicitis
endocervix
endocrine
endocrinologist
endocrinology
endocrinopathy
endogenous
endolymph
endolymphatic
endolysin
endometrial
endometrioma
endometriosis
endometritis
endometrium
endomorphic
endomorphy
endoneurium
endoparasite
end-organ
endorphin
endorse
endorsed
endorsing
endoscope
endoscopic
endoscopic retrograde
  cholangio-pancreato·
  graphy (ERCP)

endoscopy
endothelial
endothelioma
endothelium
endotoxic
endotoxin
endotracheal
end-plate
endurance
endure
endured
enduring
enema
enemata
enemies
enemy
energetic
energetically
energies
energy
enervate
enervated
enervating
enflurane
enforce
enforced
enforcement
enforcing
engage
engaged
engagement
engaging
Engerix B®
engine
engineer
English
engorged
engorgement
engross
enhance
enhanced
enhancement

enhancing
enigma
enigmatic
enigmatically
enjoy
enjoyable
enlarge
enlarged
enlarging
enlist
en masse
enmity
ennui
enormity
enormous
enough
enquire
enquired
enquirer
enquiries
enquiring
enquiry
enrage
enraged
enraging
enrol
enroll
enrolled
enrolling
enrolment
en route
ensconce
ensconced
ensconcing
ensemble
ensheathed
ensue
ensued
ensuing
ensure
ensured
ensuring

entail
entailed
entailing
Entamoeba
Entamoeba histolytica
entangle
entangled
entangling
enteric
enteritis
Enterobacteriaceae
enterobiasis
Enterobius
  vermicularis
enterocele
Enterococcus
enterocolitis
enteropathy
enterostomy
enterotoxin
enterovirus
enterprise
enterprising
enthusiasm
enthusiast
enthusiastic
enthusiastically
entire
entirely
entirety
entitle
entitled
entitling
entity
entoderm
entodermal
entomologist
entomology
Entonox®
entrails
entrance
entranced

entrancing
entrant
entrenched
entrepreneur
entries
entropion
entropy
entry
enucleate
enucleation
enumerate
enumerated
enumerating
enumeration
enuresis
envelop
envelope
enveloped
enveloping
enviable
enviably
envied
envious
environment
environmental
environmentalist
environmentally
envisage
envisaged
envisaging
envoy
envy
envying
enzymatic
enzyme
eosin
eosinophil
eosinophilia
eosinophilic
eosinophilic
  granuloma
Epanutin®

ependymoma
ephedrine
epic
epicanthal
epicanthic
epicanthus
epicardium
epicondylar
epicondyle
epicondylitis
epidemic
epidemiological
epidemiologically
epidemiologist
epidemiology
epidermal
epidermis
epidermolysis
Epidermophyton
epididymal
epididymectomy
epididymis
epididymitis
epididymo-orchitis
epidural
epigastric
epigastrium
epiglottis
epiglottitis
epilate
epilation
epilepsy
epileptic
epileptiform
epileptogenic
Epilim®
epilogue
epiloia
epilymph
epinephrine
epiphora
epiphyseal

epiphyses
epiphysis
epiphysitis
epiploic
episclera
episcleral
episcleritis
episiotomy
episode
episodic
epispadias
epistaxes
epistaxis
epistle
epitaph
epithelial
epithelialization
epithelioid
epithelioma
epithelium
epitome
epitomize
epitomized
epitomizing
epitrochlea
epitrochlear
epoch
eponym
eponymous
epoprostenol
Eppy®
Epsom salts
Epstein Barr
  virus (EBV)
Epstein's pearls
equable
equably
equal
equality
equalize
equalized
equalizing

equalled
equalling
equally
Equanil®
equanimity
equate
equated
equating
equation
equator
equatorial
equidistant
equilateral
equilibrium
equine
equinox
equinus
equip
equipped
equipping
equitable
equitably
equity
equivalent
equivocal
equivocally
equivocate
equivocated
equivocating
eradicate
eradicated
eradicating
eradication
erase
erased
eraser
erasing
Erb's palsy
erect
erectile
erection
erector

ergocalciferol
ergometer
ergometric
ergometrine
ergometry
ergonomics
ergot
ergotamine
ergotism
erode
eroded
eroding
erogenous
erosion
erosive
errand
errant
errata
erratic
erratically
erratum
erroneous
error
erthrasma
erthroderma
eructation
erupt
eruption
Erwinase®
erysipelas
erysipeloid
erythema
erythema ab igne
erythema annulare
erythema infectiosum
erythema marginatum
erythema multiforme
erythematous
erythraemia
erythrasma
erythroblast
erythroblastic

erythroblastosis fetalis
erythrocytes
erythrocytic
erythrocytosis
erythroderma
erythrogenic
erythromycin
Erythoped®
erythropoiesis
erythropoietin
erythrosine
Esbach's reagent
Esbatal®
escalate
escalated
escalating
escalation
escalator
escapade
escape
escaped
escaping
escapism
eschar
Escherichia
Escherichia coli
escort
eserine
Eskamel®
esoteric
especial
especially
espionage
esplanade
essay
essence
essential
essentially
establish
estate
esteem
ester

esterification
estimate
estimated
estimating
estimation
estolate
Estraderm®
estramustine
estranged
Estrapak®
estropipate
estuaries
estuary
etc
etch
eternal
eternally
eternity
ethacrynic acid
ethambutol
ethamivan
ethamsylate
ethanol
ethanolamine oleate
ether
ethical
ethically
ethics
ethinyloestradiol
ethionamide
ethmoid
ethmoidal
ethmoidectomy
ethnic
ethnological
ethnologically
ethnology
ethoglucid
ethosuximide
ethyl chloride
ethynodiol diacetate
etiocholanolone

etiquette
etodolac
etomidate
etoposide
etretinate
eucalypti
eucalyptus
eucalyptuses
eugenics
Euglucon®
Eugynon 30®
Eugynon 50®
Eumovate®
eunuch
euphemism
euphemistic
euphemistically
euphoria
euphoric
Eurax®
Eurax-Hydro·
  cortisone®
European
eusol
eustachian
euthanasia
euthyroid
evacuant
evacuate
evacuated
evacuating
evacuation
evade
evaded
evading
evaluate
evaluated
evaluating
evaluation
evanescent
evaporate
evaporated

evaporating
evaporation
evasion
evasive
evenness
eventful
eventfully
eventration
eventual
eventualities
eventuality
eventually
evermore
eversion
every
everybody
everyone
everything
everywhere
evict
eviction
evidence
evident
evidently
evil
evilly
evisceration
evocative
evolution
evolutionary
evolutive
evolve
evolved
evolving
evulsion
Ewing's tumour
exacerbation
exact
exacting
exaggerate
exaggerated
exaggerating

exaggeration
examination
examine
examined
examiner
examining
example
exanthem
exanthema
exanthemata
exanthematous
exasperate
exasperated
exasperating
exasperation
excavate
excavated
excavating
excavation
excavator
exceed
excel
excelled
excellence
excellent
excelling
excepting
exception
exceptional
exceptionally
excerpt
excess
excesses
excessive
excessively
exchange
exchanged
exchanging
exchequer
excise
excised
excising

excision
excitability
excitable
excitably
excitation
excitatory
excite
excited
exciting
exclaim
exclamation
exclude
excluded
excluding
exclusion
exclusive
excoriated
excoriation
excrement
excrescence
excreta
excrete
excreted
excreting
excretion
excretory
excruciating
excursion
excuse
excused
excusing
execute
executed
executing
execution
executive
executor
exemplary
exemplified
exemplify
exemplifying
exempt

exemption
exercise
exercised
exercise-induced
exercising
exert
exertion
exfoliation
exfoliative
ex gratia
exhalation
exhale
exhaust
exhaustive
exhibit
exhibition
exhibitionism
exhibitionist
exhibitor
exhilarate
exhilarated
exhilarating
exhort
exhumation
exhume
exhumed
exhuming
exigencies
exigency
exigent
exile
exiled
exiling
exist
existence
exit
exocrine
ex officio
exogenous
exomphalos
exonerate
exonerated

exonerating
exoneration
exophthalmic
exophthalmos
exorbitant
exorcism
exorcist
exoskeleton
exostosis
exotic
exotically
exotoxin
expand
expanse
expansion
expansive
expect
expectancy
expectant
expectation
expectorant
expectorate
expectoration
expediency
expedient
expedite
expedited
expediting
expedition
expel
expelled
expelling
expend
expenditure
expense
expensive
experience
experienced
experiencing
experiment
experimental
experimentally

expert
expertise
expiate
expiated
expiating
expiration
expiratory
expire
expired
expiring
expiry
explain
explanation
explanatory
expletive
explicable
explicably
explicit
explode
exploded
exploding
exploration
exploratory
explore
explored
explorer
exploring
explosion
explosive
exponent
export
exportation
expose
exposed
exposing
exposure
expression
expressive
expropriate
expropriated
expropriating
expulsion

expulsive
expurgate
expurgated
expurgating
exquisite
exsanguinate
exsanguination
extant
extempore
extend
extensible
extension
extensive
extensor
extensor carpi
  radialis brevis
extensor carpi
  radialis longus
extensor carpi
  ulnaris
extensor digiti
  minimi
extensor
  digitorum
extensor
  digitorum
  brevis
extensor
  digitorum longus
extensor
  hallucis brevis
extensor
  hallucis longus
extensor indicis
extensor
  pollicis brevis
extensor
  pollicis longus
extent
extenuating
exterior
exteriorize

exterminate
exterminated
exterminating
extermination
external
external cephalic
  version (ECV)
externalize
externally
extinct
extinction
extinguish
extinguisher
extirpation
extortion
extra-amniotic
extra-articular
extracellular
extracorporeal
extracorpuscular
extracranial
extract
extraction
extractor
extradural
extramedullary
extramural
extraneous
extra-ocular
extraordinarily
extraordinary
extraperitoneal
extrapyramidal
extrasensory
extrasystole
extrauterine
extravagance
extravagant
extravasate
extravasation
extravert
extreme

extremely
extremist
extremities
extremity
extricate
extricated
extricating
extrinsic
extrovert
extrude
extrusion
extubate
extubation
exudate
exudation
exudative
exude
exuded
exuding
eye
eyeball
eyebrow
eyed
eyeglass
eye ground
eyeing
eyelash
eyelid
eyepiece

Ff

Fabahistin®
fabric
fabricate
fabricated
fabricating
fabrication

fabulous
façade
face
faced
facet
facetious
facial
facially
facies
facile
facilitate
facilitated
facilitating
facilitation
facilities
facility
facing
facsimile
fact
faction
factor
factories
factory
factotum
facultative
faculties
faculty
fade
faded
fading
faecal
faecalith
faecal-oral
faeces
faeculent
faggot
Fahrenheit
fail
failed
failing
failure
failure to thrive

faint
faintness
fair
fairness
fait accompli
faith
faithful
faithfully
faithfulness
faithless
fake
faked
faking
falciform
fall
fallacies
fallacious
fallacy
fallen
fallible
falling
fallopian
Fallot's tetralogy
false
falsehood
falsely
falsification
falsified
falsify
falsifying
falter
falx
familial
familiar
familiarity
familiarize
familiarized
familiarizing
families
family
family planning
famine

famished
famotidine
famous
fan
fanatic
fanatical
fanatically
fanaticism
fancied
fancies
Fanconi's disease or
  syndrome
fancy
fancying
fanfare
fanned
fanning
Fansidar®
fantasies
fantastic
fantastically
fantasy
far
farad
farce
farcical
fare
fared
farewell
farinaceous
faring
farmer's lung
farther
farthest
fascia
fascial
fascicular
fasciculated
fasciculation
fasciculi
fasciculus
fasciitis

fascinate
fascinated
fascinating
fascination
fashionable
fashionably
fasten
fastidious
fastness
fat
fatal
fatalities
fatality
fatally
fate
fated
fateful
fatefully
father
father-in-law
fathers-in-law
fathom
fatigability
fatigue
fat-pad
fat-soluble
fatter
fattest
fatty
fatuous
fauces
faucet
faucial
fault
faultless
faulty
fauna
faux pas
Faverin®
favism
favour
favourable

favourably
favourite
fawn
fax machine
fear
fearful
fearfully
fearless
fearlessly
feasibility
feasible
feasibly
feast
feat
feather
feathery
feature
featured
featuring
febrile
February
fecundate
fecundation
fecundity
fed
federal
federated
federation
feeble
feebly
feed
feedback
feeder
feeding
feel
feeler
feeling
feet
Fefol®
Fehling's reagent or
solution
feign

Feldene®
feline
Felix-Weil reaction
fell
fellatio
felled
felling
fellow
fellowship
felon
felonies
felony
felt
Felty's syndrome
felypressin
female
feminine
femininity
feminism
feminist
feminization
Femodene®
femora
femoral
femoropopliteal
Femulen®
femur
fenbufen
fender
fenestra
fenestrate
fenestration
fenfluramine
fenoprofen
Fenopron®
fenoterol
fentanyl
Fentazin®
Feospan®
ferment
fermentation
ferocious

ferocity
ferric
ferried
ferries
Ferrograd®
ferrous fumarate
ferrous gluconate
ferrous glycine
 sulphate
ferrous succinate
ferrous sulphate
ferry
ferrying
fertile
fertility
fertilization
fertilize
fertilized
fertilizer
fertilizing
fervent
fester
festination
festival
festive
festivities
festivity
fetal
fetch
fête
fetid
fetish
fetishes
fetishism
fetishist
fetoplacental
fetor
fetoscopy
feud
feudal
fever
fevered

feverish
fiancé
fiancée
fibre
fibreglass
fibreoptics
fibril
fibrillar
fibrillary
fibrillated
fibrillation
fibrillolysis
fibrin
fibrinogen
fibrinolysin
fibrinolysis
fibrinolytic
fibrinous
fibroadenoma
fibroadenosis
fibroblast
fibroblastic
fibrocartilage
fibrocystic
fibrocyte
fibro-elastic
fibro-elastosis
fibroid
fibroma
fibromata
fibromatosis
fibromatous
fibromuscular
fibromyoma
fibromyomata
fibromyomatous
fibroplasia
fibrosarcoma
fibrose
fibrosing
 alveolitis
fibrosis

fibrositis
fibrotic
fibrous
fibrovascular
fibula
fibular
fickle
Fick's principle
fiction
fictitious
fidelity
fidget
field
field-marshal
fiend
fierce
fiery
fifteen
fifteenth
fifth
fiftieth
fifty
fight
fighter
fighting
figment
figurative
figure
figured
filament
filamentation
filamentous
Filaria
filarial
filariasis
filaricide
file
filed
filial
filiform
filigree
filing

Filix mas
fill
filled
filling
Filofax®
filter
filth
filthy
filtrate
filtration
filum
filum terminale
fimbria
fimbriae
fimbrial
fimbriated
fimbriation
final
finale
finality
finalization
finalize
finalized
finalizing
finally
finance
financed
financial
financially
financier
financing
find
finding
fine
fined
finery
finesse
finger
fingerprint
finger-stall
fining
finish

finite
Finnish
fiord
fire
fired
fireworks
firing
firmament
first
fiscal
fish
fisherman
fishmonger
fishy
fissile
fission
fissure
fistula
fistulae
fistular
fistulous
fitful
fitfully
fitness
fitted
fitter
fittest
fitting
fixation
fixative
fixedly
fixture
fjord
flabbergasted
flabbiness
flabby
flaccid
flaccidity
flag
flagella
flagellate
flagellation

Ff

flagellum
flagged
flagging
flagrant
Flagyl®
flail chest
flak
flake
flaked
flaking
flamboyant
flame
flamed
flaming
flammable
flange
flank
flannel
flannelette
flare
flared
flaring
flask
flat
flat-foot
flatten
flatter
flattery
flattest
flatulence
flatulent
flatus
flatworm
flaunt
flavour
flavoxate
flax
flea
flecainide
fleck
flecked
fled

fledged
fledgling
flee
fleeing
fleeting
flesh
fleshy
Fletchers' Enema®
flew
flex
flexibility
flexible
flexion
flexitime
flexor
flexor carpi radialis
flexor carpi ulnaris
flexor digiti minimi
flexor digiti minimi
    brevis
flexor digitorum
flexor digitorum brevis
flexor digitorum
    longus
flexor digitorum
    profundus
flexor hallucis brevis
flexor hallucis longus
flexor pollicis brevis
flexor pollicis longus
flexural
flexure
flick
flicker
flies
flight
flightiness
flight of ideas
flighty
flimsy
flinch
fling

flinging
flippancy
flippant
flipper
flirt
flirtation
flirtatious
float
floaters
floating kidney
flocculation
flocculent
flock
flood
flooding
floodlighting
floor
floppy
flora
floral
florid
Florinef®
florist
flotation
flour
floury
flow
flower
flowmeter
flown
Floxapen®
flu
Fluanxol®
fluclorolone acetonide
flucloxacillin
fluconazole
fluctuant
fluctuate
fluctuated
fluctuating
fluctuation
flucytosine

fludrocortisone
flue
fluency
fluent
fluffy
fluid
fluid-level
fluke
flumazenil
flung
flunisolide
flunitrazepam
fluocinolone acetonide
fluocinonide
fluocortolone
fluoresce
fluorescein
fluorescent
fluorescent
  treponemal antibody
  (FTA)
fluoridate
fluoridation
fluoride
fluoridize
fluoridized
fluoridizing
fluorometholone
fluoroscopy
fluorouracil
flupenthixol
flupenthixol decanoate
fluphenazine
flurandrenolone
flurazepam
flurbiprofen
flush
flushes
fluspirilene
flute
fluted
fluvoxamine

flux
fly
flyover
foam
focalization
foci
focus
focused
focuses
focusing
focussed
focussing
foe
foetid
foetor
foetus
foggy
foil
foist
folder
Foley catheter
foliage
folic acid
folie à deux
folinate
folinic acid
folklore
folksong
follicle
follicle-stimulating
  hormone
follicular
folliculitis
folliculosis
folliculus
follies
follow
folly
fomentation
fomite
fond
fondle

fondled
fondling
fontanelle
food
fool
foolhardy
foolish
foolishness
foolproof
foolscap
foot
footling
footprint
footstep
footwear
foramen
foramen magnum
foramen ovale
foramina
forbade
forbear
forbearing
forbid
forbidden
forbidding
forbore
force
forced
forceful
forcefully
forceps
forcible
forcibly
forcing
fore
forearm
foreboding
forebrain
forecast
forecasting
forefinger
forefront

foregone
foreground
foregut
forehead
foreign
foreigner
foreleg
foreman
foremen
foremost
forensic
foreplay
forerunner
foresaw
foresee
foreseeing
foreseen
foreshore
foresight
foreskin
forest
forestall
forestry
foretaste
foretell
foretelling
forethought
foretold
forewarn
forewaters
forfeit
forfeited
forfeiting
forgave
forgeries
forgery
forget
forgetful
forgetfully
forgetfulness
forgetting
forgive

forgiven
forgiveness
forgiving
forgo
forgoing
forgone
forgot
forgotten
formal
formaldehyde
formalin
formalities
formality
formally
format
formation
formative
former
formerly
formic
formication
formidable
formidably
formula
formulae
formulary
formulas
formulate
formulated
formulating
fornicate
fornication
fornices
fornix
forte
forthcoming
forthright
forthwith
fortieth
fortified
fortify
fortifying

fortnight
fortnightly
Fortral®
Fortran
fortress
fortresses
fortuitous
fortunate
fortunately
fortune
forty
forum
forums
forward
forwards
forwent
fosfestrol
fossa
fossae
fossil
foster
fostering
Fothergill operation
fought
foul
found
foundation
founded
founder
founding
foundling
foundries
foundry
fount
fountain
four
fourchette
Fournier's disease or
  gangrene
fourteen
fourteenth
fourth

fovea
fowl
foyer
fracas
fraction
fractional
fractionally
fractionate
fractionation
fracture
fractured
fracture-dislocation
fracturing
fragile
fragilitas
fragility
fragment
fragmentary
fragmentation
fragrant
frailties
frailty
frame
framed
framework
framing
framycetin
franc
franchise
frank
Franol®
fraternal
fraternity
fraternization
fraternize
fraternized
fraternizing
fraud
fraudulent
freckle
freedom
Freefone

freehold
freelance
freely
freeze
freezing
Freiberg's disease
   or infarction
freight
freighter
Frei test
fremitus
French
frenetic
frenetically
frenotomy
frenulum
frenum
frenzied
frequencies
frequency
frequent
fresh
freshen
Freud
Freudian
friable
Friar's balsam
friction
Friday
fridge
fried
Friedlaender's bacillus
Friedreich's ataxia
friend
friendliness
friendly
friendship
frighten
frightful
frightfully
frigid
frigidity

frill
Frisium®
frizzy
Froben®
frogman
frogmen
Frohlich's syndrome
frolic
frolicked
frolicking
front
frontage
frontal
frontalis
frontier
frostbite
frosted
frostily
frosty
froth
frothy
frown
froze
frozen
fructose
fruiterer
fruitful
fruitfully
fruition
fruitless
Frumil®
frusemide
Frusene®
frustrate
frustrated
frustrating
frustration
fry
frying
Fucidin®
fuel
fugitive

fugue
Fulcin®
fulfil
fulfilled
fulfilling
fulfilment
Fuller's earth
fullness
full-term
fully
fulminant
fulminating
fume
fumed
fumigate
fumigated
fumigating
fumigation
fuming
function
functional
functionally
functioned
functioning
fundal
fundamental
fundamentally
fundi
fundoplication
fundus
funduscopy
funeral
fungal
fungate
fungating
fungi
fungicidal
fungicide
Fungilin®
fungistatic
fungus
funguses

funiculitis
funiculus
funnel
funnel chest
funnily
funny
Furadantin®
furbish
furfur
furious
furnace
furnish
furnishings
furniture
furor
furred
furrow
furry
further
furthermore
furthest
furtive
furuncle
furuncular
furunuculosis
fury
fuse
fused
fusidate
fusidic acid
fusiform
fusing
fusion
futile
future
Fybogel®

Gg

gaberdine
gable
gadget
Gaelic
gaiety
gaily
gain
gait
galactagogue
galactase
galactocele
galactokinase
galactorrhoea
galactosaemia
galactosaemic
galactose
galaxies
galaxy
gale
gall
gallamine
gallant
gall-bladder
galleries
gallery
galley
galling
gallipot
gallon
gallop
galloped
galloping
gallows traction
gallstone
galore
galvanize
galvanized

Gg

galvanizing
galvanometer
Gamanil®
gambit
gamble
gambled
gambling
gamekeeper
gamete
gametocyte
gametogenesis
gametogensis
gamgee
gaming
gamma
gamma benzene
  hexachloride
gamma globulin
gammaglobulin
gamma ray
gammon
Ganciclovir
Ganda®
gander
ganglia
ganglioma
ganglion
ganglionate
ganglion-blocking
ganglionectomy
ganglionic
gangliosidosis
gangrene
gangrenous
gangster
gangway
Ganser syndrome
gantries
gantry
gaol
gaoler
gape

gaped
gaping
garage
garaged
garaging
garbage
garden
gardener
Gardnerella vaginalis
gargantuan
gargle
gargled
gargling
gargoylism
garlic
garment
garrison
garrotte
garrotted
garrotting
gas
gaseous
gases
gas-gangrene
gash
gashes
gasometer
gassed
Gasserian ganglion
gassing
gastrectomy
gastric
gastrin
gastritis
gastrocnemius
gastrocolic
Gastrocote®
gastroduodenal
gastroduodenostomy
gastroenteritis
gastroenterological
gastroenterologically

gastroenterology
gastroenterostomy
Gastrografin®
gastro-intestinal
gastrojejunal
gastrojejunostomy
gastro-oesophageal
gastroscope
gastroscopic
gastroscopy
gastrostomy
gastrula
gatecrash
gather
gathering
gauche
Gaucher's disease
gauge
gauged
gauging
gaunt
gauze
gave
Gaviscon®
gay
gaze
gazed
gazetteer
gazing
gear
geese
Geiger counter
gel
gelatin
gelatine
gelatinous
gem
gemellus
gemeprost
gemfibrozil
gender
gene

77

Gg

genealogies
genealogy
genera
general
generalization
generalize
generalized
generalizing
generally
generate
generated
generating
generation
generative
generator
generic
generosity
generous
genesis
genetic
genetically
geneticist
genetics
genial
genially
genicular
geniculate
geniculum
genioglossal
genioglossus
genital
genitalia
genitofemoral
genitourinary
genius
geniuses
genome
genotype
gentamicin
gentian
Genticin®
Gentisone HC®

gentle
gentleman
gentlemen
gently
gentry
genu
genuflex
genuine
genus
genu valgum
genu varum
geographical
geographically
geography
geological
geologically
geologist
geology
geometric
geometrically
geometry
geriatric
geriatrician
geriatrics
germ
German
germane
germicidal
germicide
germinal
germinate
germinated
germinating
germination
germinative
gerontological
gerontology
gesalt
gestaltism
gestation
gestational
gesticulate

gesticulated
gesticulating
gesticulation
gestodene
gestronol
gesture
gestured
gesturing
get
getting
geyser
ghastliness
ghastly
Ghon focus
Giardia
Giardia lamblia
giardiasis
gibbous
gibbus
giddiness
giddy
Giemsa stain
gifted
gigantic
gigantism
Gilbert's syndrome
gill
Gilles de la Tourette
  disease or syndrome
Gilliam's operation
gilt
gilt-edged
gimmick
ginger
gingham
gingiva
gingival
gingivectomy
gingivitis
gipsies
gipsy
gird

girder
girdle
girlhood
giro
girth
gist
give
given
giving
glabella
glabellar
glad
glamorous
glamour
glance
glanced
glancing
gland
glanders
glandular
glans
glare
glared
glaring
glass
glasses
glassily
glassy
glaucoma
glaucomatous
glaze
glazed
glazing
glenohumeral
glenoid
glia
glial
glib
glibenclamide
Glibenese®
glibness
gliclazide

glide
glided
glider
gliding
glimpse
glimpsed
glimpsing
glint
glioblastoma
  multiforme
glioma
gliomata
gliomatosis
gliomatous
gliomyoma
gliomyomata
gliosis
glipizide
gliquidone
glisten
glitter
gloat
global
globally
globe
globin
globular
globule
globulin
globus hystericus
globus pallidus
glomerular
glomerular filtration
glomerular filtration
  rate (GFR)
glomeruli
glomerulitis
glomerulonephritis
glomerulosclerosis
glomerulosclerotic
glomerulus
glomus

gloom
gloomily
gloomy
glories
glorified
glorify
glorifying
glorious
glory
glossaries
glossary
glossectomy
glossitis
glossopharyngeal
glottic
glottis
glottitis
glove
glow
glucagon
glucocorticoid
glucogenesis
gluconate
gluconeogenesis
Glucophage®
glucose
glucose 6-phosphate
  dehydrogenase
glucuronic acid
glue
glued
glue ear
gluing
Glurenorm®
glutamic
glutamic oxaloacetic
  transaminase
glutamic pyruvic
  transaminase
glutaminase
glutaraldehyde
Glutarol®

Gg

gluteal
gluten
gluten enteropathy
gluten-free
gluteus
glutinous
glycerin
glycerine
glycerin thymol
glycerol
glyceryl trinitrate
glycine
glycogen
glycogenase
glycogenesis
glycogenolysis
glycol
glycolysis
glycolytic
glycoprotein
glycopyrronium
  bromide
glycoside
glycosuria
glymidine
gnarled
gnash
gnat
gnaw
goad
go-ahead
goat
gobble
gobbled
gobbling
goblet
godfather
godliness
godmother
goggles
going
goitre

goitrogens
gold
golden
Golgi's apparatus
gonad
gonadal
gonadorelin
gonadotrophic
gonadotrophin
gonadotrophin-
  releasing
Gondafon®
gone
gong
goniometer
gonioscope
gonioscopy
goniotomy
gonococcal
gonococci
Gonococcus
gonorrhoea
gonorrhoeal
good
goodbye
good-day
goodness
Goodpasture
  syndrome
goodwill
goose
goose-pimples
gore
gored
gorgeous
goring
gory
goserelin
gospel
gossip
got
gouge

gouged
gouging
gout
gouty
govern
governess
governesses
government
governor
gown
Graafian follicle
grab
grabbed
grabbing
grace
graced
graceful
gracefully
gracilis
gracing
gracious
gradation
grade
graded
gradient
grading
gradual
gradually
graduate
graduated
graduating
graduation
graffiti
graft
grain
gram
grammar
grammatical
grammatically
gramme
Gram-negative
gramophone

Gram-positive
Gram's stain
grand
grandchild
grandchildren
grand-daughter
grandfather
grand mal
grandmother
grandson
granite
grannies
granny
grant
Granuflex®
granular
granulate
granulation
granule
granulocyte
granulocytopenia
granulocytosis
granuloma
granuloma annulare
granuloma inguinale
granulomatosis
granulomatous
graph
graphaesthesia
graphic
graphite
grasp
grass
grasses
grassy
grateful
gratefully
grater
gratification
gratified
gratify
gratifying

grating
gratis
gratitude
gratuities
gratuitous
gratuity
grave
gravel
Graves' disease
gravid
gravitation
gravitational
gravity
gravy
gray
graze
grazed
grazing
grease
greased
greasing
greasy
great
greatness
greed
greedily
greediness
greedy
Greek
green
greenery
greengrocer
greenhouse
greenish
greenness
greenstick fracture
greetings
gregarious
Gregory's mixture
grew
grey
grid

grief
grievance
grieve
grieved
grieving
grievous
Griffith's types
grill
grille
grim
grimace
grimaced
grimacing
grime
grimness
grin
grind
grinder
grinding
grinned
grinning
grip
gripe
gripped
gripping
griseofulvin
grisovin
gristle
gristly
grit
gritted
gritting
grizzled
groan
grocer
groceries
grocery
groggily
groggy
groin
grommet
groom

groove
grope
groped
groping
gross
grotesque
ground
grounded
grounding
groundless
groundwork
group
grouse
groused
grouses
grousing
grow
growing
growl
grown
growth
gruelling
gruesome
gruff
grumble
grumbled
grumbling
grunt
guanethidine
guanine
guar
guarantee
guaranteed
guaranteeing
guarantor
guard
guardian
guar gum
gubernaculum
guess
guesses
guest

guidance
guide
guidebook
guided
guiding
guild
guile
guileless
Guillain-Barré
  syndrome
guillotine
guillotined
guillotining
guilt
guiltily
guilty
guinea
guinea-pig
Guinea worm
guise
guitar
gullet
gullible
gullibly
gum
gumboil
gumma
gummata
gummatous
gummed
gumming
gumption
gun
gunned
gunning
gurgle
gurgled
gurgling
gush
gusset
gustation
gustatory

gustily
gusty
gut
Guthrie test
guts
gutta
guttae
guttate
gutted
gutter
gutting
guttural
gutturally
gym
gymnasia
gymnasium
gymnasiums
gymnast
gymnastics
gynaecological
gynaecologist
gynaecology
gynaecomastia
Gyno-Daktarin®
Gynol II®
Gyno-Pevaryl®
Gynovlar 21®
gypsies
Gypsona®
gypsum
gypsy
gyrate
gyrated
gyrating
gyratory
gyrus

Hh

H$_2$ antagonist
habit
habitable
habitat
habitation
habitual
habitually
habituation
hackles
hacksaw
had
haddock
Haelan®
haem
haemachromatosis
haemagglutination
haemagglutinin
haemangioma
haemangiomata
haemangiomatosis
haemarthroses
haemarthrosis
haematemesis
haematin
haematinic
haematite
haematocele
haematocolpos
haematocrit
haematogenous
haematological
haematologically
haematologist
haematology
haematoma
haematomata
haematomatous
haematopoiesis

haematoporphyrin
haematospermia
haematuria
haemochromatosis
haemoconcentration
haemodialysis
haemodilution
haemodynamics
haemoglobin
haemoglobinometer
haemoglobinopathy
haemoglobinuria
haemolysin
haemolysis
haemolytic
haemolyze
haemoperfusion
haemopericardium
haemoperitoneum
haemophilia
haemophiliac
Haemophilus
Haemophilus ducreyi
Haemophilus
  influenzae
haemopneumothorax
haemopoiesis
haemopoietic
haemoptyses
haemoptysis
haemorrhage
haemorrhaged
haemorrhagic
haemorrhaging
haemorrhoidal
haemorrhoidectomy
haemorrhoid
haemosiderosis
haemospermia
haemostasis
haemostatic
haemothorax

Hageman factor
Haig Ferguson
  forceps
hailstone
hairdresser
hair-raising
hairy
halcinonide
Halcion®
hale
half
half-life
halfpennies
halfpenny
halibut-liver
halitosis
hall
hallmark
hallo
Hallowe'en
hallucinate
hallucinated
hallucinating
hallucination
hallucinogens
hallucinosis
hallux
hallux rigidus
hallux valgus
hallux varus
halo
halogen
haloperidol
halothane
halt
halter
halting
halve
halved
halves
halving
hamamelis

hamartoma
Hamman-Rich
  syndrome
hammer
hammer toe
hammock
hamper
hamstring
hamstringing
hamstrung
hand
handbag
handful
handfuls
handicap
handicapped
handicraft
handiness
handiwork
handkerchief
handkerchiefs
handkerchieves
handle
handled
handling
Hand-Schüller-
  Christian disease
handsome
handwriting
handyman
hang
hangar
hanged
hanger
hanger-on
hangers-on
hanging
hangover
hanker
hankered
hankering
hankie

hankies
hanky
Hansen's disease
haphazard
haploid
happen
happened
happening
happier
happiest
happily
happiness
happy
haptoglobin
harass
harassed
harassing
harassment
harbour
hard
harden
hardily
hardiness
hardly
hardness
hardware
hardy
hare-lip
harm
harmful
harmfully
harmless
Harmogen®
harmony
harness
harnesses
harp
Harrison's sulcus
harrowing
harsh
harshness
Hartmann's solution

Hartnup disease
Harveian
harvest
harvester
Hashimoto's disease
hashish
hassle
haste
hasten
hastily
hasty
hat
hatch
hatcheries
hatchery
hatches
hatchway
hate
hated
hateful
hatefully
hating
hatred
haul
haulage
haunch
haunches
haunt
haustral
haustration
haustrum
have
haven
having
havoc
hay fever
Haymine®
haywire
hazard
hazardous
haze
hazily

hazy
head
headache
head-dress
heading
headlight
headline
headmaster
headmistress
headmistresses
headquarters
headstrong
headway
Heaf test
heal
health
healthily
healthy
heap
hear
heard
hearing
hearing aid
hearsay
hearse
heart
heart block
heartburn
hearten
heartfelt
hearth
heartily
heartless
heart-lung
hearty
heat
heath
heather
heave
heaved
heaven
heavier

heaviest
heavily
heaviness
heaving
heavy
hebephrenia
hebephrenic
Heberden's nodes
hectare
hectic
hectically
he'd
hedge
hedged
hedging
hedonism
heed
heedless
heel
hefty
height
heighten
Heimlich's manoeuvre
heinous
Heinz body
heir
heiress
heiresses
held
helicopter
helium
helix
he'll
Heller's operation
hello
helm
helmet
helminth
helminthic
helpful
helpfully
helpfulness

helping
helpless
helplessness
hemianaesthesia
hemianalgesia
hemianopia
hemiatrophy
hemicolectomy
hemidiaphragm
hemiglossectomy
Heminevrin®
hemiparesis
hemiplegia
hemiplegic
hemisphere
hemithorax
hemivertebra
hemlock
hemp
henceforth
henna
Henoch-Schönlein
  purpura
hepar
heparin
heparinize
heparinized
hepatectomize
hepatectomy
hepatic
hepatitis
hepatization
hepatocellular
hepatolenticular
hepatoma
hepatomata
hepatomegaly
hepatosplenomegaly
hepatotoxic
hepatotoxicity
hepatotoxin
heptagon

Hh

heptagonal
herald
herb
herbaceous
herbal
herbalist
herbivore
herbivorous
herd
here
hereabouts
hereafter
hereby
hereditary
heredity
herewith
heritage
hermaphrodism
hermaphrodite
hermetically
hernia
hernial
herniate
herniation
hernioplasty
herniorrhaphy
herniotomy
hero
heroes
heroic
heroically
heroin
heroine
heroism
herpangina
herpes
Herpes labialis
Herpes simplex
herpetic
herpetiform
Herpid®
hers

hertz
Herxheimer reaction
he's
hesitancy
hesitant
hesitate
hesitated
hesitating
hesitation
Hess test
hetastarch
heterogenous
heterologous
heteroplasty
heterosexual
heterozygote
heterozygous
hew
hewed
hewing
hewn
hexacetonide
hexachlorophane
hexagon
hexagonal
hexamine
hexanoate
hexetidine
Hexopal®
hexose
hiatal
hiatus
hibernate
hibernated
hibernating
hibernation
Hibiscrub®
Hibitane®
hiccup
hid
hidden
hide

hideous
hiding
hidradenitis
hidradenitis
  suppurativa
hidrosis
hierarchy
hieroglyphics
hi-fi
high
high density
  lipoprotein
higher
highest
high fidelity
highlight
highly
highness
high-risk
highway
hijack
hijacker
hike
hiked
hiking
hilar
hilarious
hilarity
hili
hilum
hind
hind-brain
hinder
hindmost
hindrance
hindsight
hinge
hinged
hinging
hint
hippocampal
hippocampus

hippocratic
hire
hired
hire purchase
hiring
Hirschsprung's
  disease
hirsute
hirsutism
Hismanal®
hiss
hisses
histamine
histamine H_1
  -receptor
histamine H_2
  -receptor
histidinaemia
histidine
histiocytes
histiocytoma
histiocytosis
histiocytosis X
histochemistry
histocompatibility
histological
histologically
histology
histopathology
Histoplasma
histoplasmosis
historian
historic
historical
historically
histories
history
histrionic
Histryl®
hit
hitch
hitches

hitchhike
hitchhiked
hitchhiking
hither
hitherto
hitting
hive
hoard
hoarse
hoarseness
hoax
hoaxes
hobbies
hobby
hockey
Hodge's pessary
Hodgkin's disease
hoe
hoed
hoeing
hoist
hold
holdall
holder
holding
hold-up
hole
holiday
holiness
holistic
Hollister®
hollow
holly
Holmes-Adie
  syndrome
holy
homage
Homans' sign
homatropine
home
homed
homeliness

homely
homeopathic
homeopathy
homeostasis
homesick
homewards
homework
homicidal
homicide
homing
homocystine
homocystinuria
homoeopath
homogeneous
homogenization
homogenize
homogenized
homogenizing
homogenous
homograft
homologous
homologue
homonym
homonymous
homosexual
homosexuality
homozygote
homozygous
homunculus
honest
honesty
honey
honorarium
honorary
honour
honourable
honourably
hoof
hoofs
hook
hookworm
hooligan

hooves
hop
hope
hoped
hopeful
hopefully
hopefulness
hopeless
hopelessness
hoping
hopped
hopping
hopscotch
horde
horizon
horizontal
hormone
hormonogenesis
Horner syndrome
hornet
horny
horrendous
horrible
horribly
horrid
horrified
horrify
horrifying
horror
horsepower
horseshoe
horticultural
horticulture
horticulturist
hose
hosiery
hospitable
hospitably
hospital
hospitality
hospitalization
hospitalize

host
hostage
hostel
hostelries
hostelry
hostess
hostesses
hostile
hostilities
hostility
hot
hothouse
hotter
hottest
hound
hour
hour-glass contraction
hourly
house
housed
household
householder
housekeeper
housemaid's knee
housewife
housing
hover
hovercraft
Howell-Jolly bodies
however
huddle
huddled
huddling
hue
hug
huge
hugged
hugging
hulk
hull
hullo
hum

human
Human Actraphane®
Human Actrapid®
Human Actrapid
  Penfill®
human chorionic
  gonadotrophin
  (HCG)
humane
human immuno·
  deficiency virus (HIV)
Human Initard 50/50®
Human Insulatard®
humanism
humanist
humanitarian
humanity
humanized
Human Mixtard
  30/70®
Human Monotard®
human placental
  lactogen
Human Protaphane®
human T-cell
  lymphotropic virus
Human Ultratard®
Human Velosulin®
humble
humbly
humeral
humeri
humerus
humid
humidifier
humidity
humiliate
humiliated
humiliating
humiliation
humility
hummed

humming
humor
humoral immunity
humorist
humorous
humour
hump
humpbacked
Humulin 1®
Humulin M1®
Humulin M2®
Humulin M3®
Humulin M4®
Humulin S®
Humulin Zn®
humus
hunch
hunchback
hunches
hundred
hundredth
hundredweight
hung
Hungarian
Hungary
hunger
hungrily
hungry
Hunter-Hurler
  syndrome
Hunter syndrome
Huntington's chorea
Hurler syndrome
hurricane
hurried
hurry
hurrying
hurt
hurtful
hurtfully
husband
husk

hutch
hutches
Hutchinson's teeth
hyalin
hyaline
hyaline membrane
  disease
hyalinization
hyaluronidase
hybrid
hybridization
Hycal®
hydatid cyst
hydatidiform
Hydergine®
hydralazine
hydramnios
hydrant
hydrate
hydration
hydraulic
hydro
hydrobromide
hydrocarbon
hydrocele
hydrocephalic
hydrocephalus
hydrocephaly
hydrochlorothiazide
hydrocolloid
hydrocortisone
hydroelectric
hydroflumethiazide
hydrogel
hydrogen
hydrogenase
hydrogenate
hydrogenation
hydrogen peroxide
hydrolyse
hydrolysis
hydrolytic

hydrometer
hydronephrosis
hydropathic
hydrophobia
hydrophylic
hydropneumothorax
hydrops
hydrops foetalis
hydrosalpinx
hydrotalcite
hydrotherapy
hydrothorax
hydroureter
hydrous
hydroxocobalamin
hydroxyapatite
hydroxychloroquine
hydroxycholecalciferol
hydroxyprogesterone
hexanoate
hydroxyquinoline
hydroxyurea
hydroxyzine
hygiene
hygienic
hygienically
hygienist
hygroma
hygromata
hygromatous
hygrometer
hygroscopic
Hygroton®
hymen
hymenectomy
hymenotomy
hyoid
hyoscine butylbromide
hyperacidity
hyperactive
hyperactivity
hyperacusis

Hh

hyperacute
hyperadrenalism
hyperaemia
hyperaemic
hyperaesthesia
hyperaesthetic
hyperaldosteronism
hyperalgesia
hyperalimentation
hyperbaric oxygen
hyperbilirubinaemia
hyperbilirubinaemic
hypercalcaemia
hypercalcaemic
hypercalciuria
hypercapnia
hypercapnic
hyperchloraemic
hyperchlorhydria
hyperchlorhydric
hypercholesterol·
  aemia
hypercholesterolaemic
hyperemesis
hyperextend
hyperextension
hyperflexion
hyperglycaemia
hyperglycaemic
hypergonadism
hyperhidrosis
hyperinsulinism
hyperkalaemia
hyperkalaemic
hyperkeratose
hyperkeratosis
hyperkeratotic
hyperkinesis
hyperkinetic
hyperlipidaemia
hyperlipoproteinaemia
hypermagnesaemia

hypermarket
hypermetropia
hypermetropic
hypermobility
hypermotility
hypernatraemia
hypernatraemic
hypernephroma
hypernephromata
hyperosmolar diabetic
  coma
hyperosmolarity
hyperosmolar
  nonketotic
hyperostosis
hyperparathyroidism
hyperphosphataemia
hyperphosphataemic
hyperpigmentation
hyperpituitarism
hyperplasia
hyperplastic
hyperpyrexia
hyperpyrexial
hyper-reflexia
hypersalivation
hypersecretion
hypersensitive
hypersensitivity
hypersensitization
hypersexuality
hypersplenism
hypertelorism
hypertension
hypertensive
hyperthermia
hyperthermic
hyperthyroid
hyperthyroidism
hypertonia
hypertonic
hypertonicity

hypertrichosis
hypertrophic
hypertrophy
hyperuricaemia
hyperuricaemic
hyperventilation
hypervitaminosis
hypervolaemia
hypha
hyphae
hyphaema
hyphen
hypnagogic
hypnosis
hypnotherapy
hypnotic
hypnotism
hypnotist
hypnotize
hypnotized
hypnotizing
hypo-aesthesia
hypo-albuminaemia
hypo-calcaemia
hypocalcaemic
hypocapnia
hypochloraemia
hypochloraemic
hypochlorhydria
hypochlorite
hypochondria
hypochondriac
hypochondriacal
hypochondriasis
hypochondrium
hypochromia
hypochromic
hypocrisy
hypocrite
hypocritical
hypocritically
hypodermic

hypofunction
hypogammaglobulin·
  aemia
hypogammaglobulin·
  aemic
hypogastric
hypogastrium
hypoglossal
hypoglycaemia
hypoglycaemic
hypogonadism
hypokalaemia
hypokalaemic
hypokinesis
hypokinetic
hypomagnesaemia
hypomagnesaemic
hypomania
hypomanic
hyponatraemia
hyponatraemic
hypo-osmolarity
hypoparathyroidism
hypopharynx
hypophosphataemia
hypophosphataemic
hypophyseal
hypophysectomize
hypophysectomy
hypophysis
hypopigmentation
hypopituitarism
hypoplasia
hypoplastic
hypoproteinaemia
hypoproteinaemic
hypopyon
hyposecretion
hyposensitivity
hyposensitization
hypospadias

hypostasis
hypostatic
hypotension
hypotensive
hypothalamic
hypothalamus
hypothenar eminence
hypothermia
hypotheses
hypothesis
hypothetical
hypothetically
hypothyroid
hypothyroidism
hypotonia
hypotonic
hypotonicity
hypoventilation
hypovitaminaemia
hypovitaminosis
hypovolaemia
hypovolaemic
hypoxaemia
hypoxaemic
hypoxia
hypoxic
hypromellose
hypsarrhythmia
Hypurin Isophane®
Hypurin Lente®
Hypurin Neutral®
Hypurin Protamine
  Zinc®
Hypurin Soluble®
hysterectomy
hysteria
hysteric
hysterical
hysterically
hysterics
hysterosalpingectomy

hysterosalpingo·
  graphy
hysterotomy

Ii

iatrogenic
ibuprofen
ice cream
ichthammol
Ichthopaste®
ichthyoses
ichthyosis
icicle
icily
icing
icteric
icterus
icy
I'd
id
idea
ideal
idealism
idealist
ideally
ideation
identical
identically
identification
identified
identify
identifying
identities
identity
ideomotor
idiocies
idiocy

idiom
idiopathic
idiosyncrasies
idiosyncrasy
idiosyncratic
idiosyncratically
idiot
idiotic
idiotically
idioventricular
idle
idled
idleness
idling
idly
idoxuridine
Iduridin®
ifosfamide
ignite
ignited
igniting
ignition
ignominious
ignorance
ignorant
ignore
ignored
ignoring
ileac
ileal
ileal bladder
ileal conduit
ileitis
ileocaecal
ileocolic
ileostomy
ileoureterostomy
ileum
ileus
iliac
iliacus
Iliadin-Mini®

iliofemoral
iliopsoas
iliotibial tract
ilium
I'll
ill
illegal
illegally
illegibility
illegible
illegibly
illegitimacy
illegitimate
illicit
illiteracy
illiterate
illness
illnesses
illogical
illogically
illumination
illusion
illusional
illustrate
illustrated
illustrating
illustration
illustrative
illustrator
I'm
image
image-intensifier
imagery
imaginary
imagination
imaginative
imagine
imagined
imagining
imbalance
imbecile
imbue

imbued
imbuing
Imferon®
imidazole
imipenem
imipramine
imitate
imitated
imitating
imitation
immaculate
immaterial
immature
immediacy
immediate
immediately
immemorial
immense
immensity
immerse
immersed
immersing
immersion
immigrant
immigration
imminent
immobile
immobility
immobilization
immobilize
immobilized
immobilizing
immoderate
immoral
immovable
immovably
immune
immunity
immunization
immunize
immunized
immunizing

immunoassay
immunocompromised
immunodeficiency
immunofluorescence
immunogenesis
immunogenetic
immunogenicity
immunoglobulin
immunological
immunologically
immunologist
immunology
immunostimulant
immunosuppressant
immunosuppressed
immunosuppression
immunosuppressive
Imodium®
impact
impacted
impaction
impaired
impairment
impale
impaled
impaling
impalpable
impart
impartial
impartiality
impartially
impassable
impasse
impassive
impatience
impatient
impeccable
impeccably
impedance
impede
impeded
impediment

impeding
impending
imperative
imperceptible
imperceptibly
imperfect
imperfection
imperforate
impermeable
impersonal
impersonally
impersonate
impersonated
impersonating
impersonation
impertinence
impertinent
imperturbable
impervious
impetiginous
impetigo
impetuosity
impetuous
impetus
impinge
impinged
impinging
implant
implantation
implement
implicate
implicated
implicating
implication
implicit
implied
imply
implying
impolite
import
importance
important

impose
imposed
imposing
imposition
impossibility
impossible
impossibly
impostor
impotence
impotent
impound
impoverish
impracticability
impracticable
impracticably
impractical
impracticality
impractically
impregnable
impregnate
impressed
impression
impressionable
impressive
imprint
imprinting
improbability
improbable
improbably
impromptu
improper
improprieties
impropriety
improve
improved
improving
improvisation
improvise
improvised
improvising
impudence
impudent

impulse
impulsion
impulsive
impunity
impure
impurities
impurity
Imunovir®
Imuran®
inability
inaccessibility
inaccessible
inaccessibly
inaccurate
inaction
inactivate
inactivation
inactive
inactivity
inadequacies
inadequacy
inadequate
inadequately
inadmissible
inadvertent
inane
inanimate
inapplicable
inappropriate
inarticulate
inasmuch as
inassimilable
inattention
inaudible
inaudibly
inaugural
inaugurate
inaugurated
inaugurating
inauguration
inauspicious
inborn

inbred
inbreeding
incalculable
incapable
incapacitate
incapacitated
incapacitating
incapacity
incarcerated
incense
incensed
incensing
incentive
inception
incessant
incest
inch
inches
incidence
incident
incidental
incidentally
incineration
incinerator
incipient
incise
incised
incision
incisional
incisive
incisor
incite
incited
inciting
incivilities
incivility
inclination
incline
inclined
inclining
include
included

including
inclusion
inclusion bodies
inclusive
incognito
incoherent
incombustible
income
incoming
incommunicado
incomparable
incomparably
incompatibility
incompatible
incompetence
incompetent
incomplete abortion
incomprehensible
incomprehensibly
incomprehension
inconceivable
inconceivably
inconclusive
incongruity
incongruous
inconsequential
inconsequentially
inconsiderable
inconsiderate
inconsistency
inconsistent
inconspicuous
inconstant
incontinence
incontinent
incontrovertible
incontrovertibly
inconvenience
inconvenient
incoordination
incorporate
incorporated

incorporating
incorrect
incorrigible
incorrigibly
incorruptible
increase
increased
increasing
incredibility
incredible
incredibly
incredulity
incredulous
increment
incriminate
incriminated
incriminating
incubate
incubated
incubating
incubation
incubator
incumbent
incur
incurable
incurably
incurred
incurring
incus
indapamide
indebted
indecency
indecent
indecision
indecisive
indeed
indefatigable
indefatigably
indefensible
indefensibly
indefinable
indefinably

indefinite
indefinitely
indelible
indelibly
indemnity
indent
indentation
independence
independent
Inderal®
Inderetic®
Inderex®
indescribable
indescribably
indestructible
indeterminate
index
indexes
Indian
indicant
indicate
indicated
indicating
indication
indicative
indicator
indices
indict
indictment
indifference
indifferent
indigenous
indigestible
indigestion
indignant
indignation
indignities
indignity
indirect
indiscretion
indiscriminate
indispensable

indispensably
indisposed
indisposition
indisputable
indisputably
indistinct
indistinguishable
indistinguishably
individual
individualist
individuality
individually
indivisible
Indocid®
indole
indolent
indomethacin
indomitable
indomitably
indoor
indoramin
induce
induced
induced abortion
inducer
inducing
induct
inductance
induction
inductive
indulge
indulged
indulgence
indulging
indurated
induration
industrial
industrialist
industrious
inebriated
inedible
ineffective

ineffectual
ineffectually
inefficiency
inefficient
ineligibility
ineligible
ineptitude
inequalities
inequality
inert
inertia
inescapable
inescapably
inestimable
inestimably
inevitability
inevitable
inevitable abortion
inevitably
inexcusable
inexcusably
inexhaustible
inexpensive
inexperience
inexperienced
inexplicable
inexplicably
inexpressible
inexpressibly
in extremis
inextricable
inextricably
Infacol®
infallible
infallibly
infamous
infancy
infant
infanticide
infantile
infantilism
infarct

infarction
infect
infection
infectious
infective
infectivity
infer
inference
inferior
inferiority
infernal
infernally
inferolateral
inferred
inferring
infertile
infertility
infest
infestation
infested
infiltrate
infiltration
infinite
infinitesimal
infinitesimally
infinitive
infirm
infirmaries
infirmary
infirmities
infirmity
inflammable
inflammation
inflammatory
inflate
inflated
inflating
inflation
inflationary
inflator
inflexible
inflict

influence
influenced
influencing
influential
influentially
influenza
influenzal
Influvac®
influx
inform
informal
informality
informally
informant
information
informative
informer
infra-mammary
infra-orbital
infra-red
infundibula
infundibular
infundibulum
infuriate
infuriated
infuriating
infusion
ingenious
ingenuity
ingestion
ingrained
ingratitude
ingredient
ingrowing
inguinal
inhabit
inhabitant
inhalant
inhalation
inhalational
inhale
inhaled

inhaler
inhaling
inherent
inherit
inheritance
inhibit
inhibited
inhibiting
inhibition
inhibitor
inhibitory
inhospitable
inhospitably
inhuman
inhumane
Initard 50/50®
initial
initialled
initialling
initially
initiate
initiated
initiating
initiation
initiative
initiator
inject
injected
injection
injector
injure
injured
injuries
injuring
injury
injustice
inland
inmate
inmost
innate
inner
innervation

innings
innocence
innocent
innocuous
innominate
Innovace®
innovation
innuendo
innuendoes
innumerable
innumeracy
innumerate
inoculable
inoculate
inoculated
inoculating
inoculation
inoculator
inoculum
inoffensive
inoperable
inopportune
inordinate
inorganic
inosine pranobex
inosital®
inotropic
in-patient
inplantation
input
inquest
inquire
inquired
inquirer
inquiries
inquiring
inquiry
inquisition
inquisitive
insane
insanitary
insanity

insatiable
insatiably
inscription
inscrutable
inscrutably
insect
Insecta
insecticidal
insecticide
insectivore
insecure
insecurity
insemination
insensibility
insensible
insensitive
inseparable
inseparably
insert
insertion
inset
inside
insidious
insight
insignificance
insignificant
insincere
insincerity
insinuate
insinuated
insinuating
insinuation
insist
insistence
insistent
in situ
insolation
insolubility
insoluble
insomnia
insomniac
inspect

inspection
inspector
inspiration
inspiratory
inspire
inspissate
inspissated
instability
instal
install
installation
installed
installing
instalment
instance
instant
instantaneous
instead
instep
instigate
instigated
instigating
instigation
instil
instillation
instilled
instilling
instinct
instinctive
instinctively
institute
instituted
instituting
institution
institutional
institutionalization
instruct
instruction
instructive
instructor
instrument
instrumental

instrumentation
insubordinate
insubordination
insufferable
insufferably
insufficiency
insufficient
insufflation
insufflator
Insulatard®
insulate
insulated
insulating
insulation
insulin
insulinoma
insuperable
insuperably
insurance
insure
insured
insuring
insurmountable
insurmountably
insusceptibility
intact
intake
Intal®
intangible
intangibly
integral
integrate
integrated
integrating
integration
Integrin®
integrity
intellect
intellectual
intelligence
intelligent
intelligible

intelligibly
intemperance
intemperate
intend
intense
intensification
intensified
intensifier
intensify
intensifying
intensity
intensive
intent
intention
intentionally
inter
interact
interaction
inter alia
interalveolar
interarticular
interatrial
intercede
interceded
interceding
intercellular
intercept
intercerebral
intercession
interchange
interchangeable
interchanged
interchanging
intercom
intercostal
intercourse
intercurrent
interdigital
interdigitation
interest
interesting
interface

interfere
interfered
interference
interfering
interferon
interim
interlobular
interlock
intermarriage
intermediaries
intermediary
intermediate
intermenstrual
interment
interminable
interminably
intermittent
intern
internal
internally
international
internationally
internist
interosseal
interossei
interosseous
interphalangeal
interphase
interpolated
interpolation
interpret
interpretation
interred
interring
interrupt
interruption
interruptus
intersection
intersex
interspace
intersperse
interspersed

interspersing
interspinous
interstices
interstitial
interstitial cell of
  Leydig
intertrigenous
intertrigo
intertrochanteric
interval
intervene
intervened
intervening
intervention
interventricular
intervertebral
interview
intestinal
intestine
intima
intimacy
intimal
intimate
intimated
intimating
intimation
in-toeing
intolerable
intolerably
intolerance
intonation
intone
intoned
intoning
intoxicant
intoxicate
intoxicated
intoxicating
intoxication
intra-abdominal
intra-amniotic
intra-arterial

intra-arterially
intra-articular
intra-atrial
intracapsular
intracardiac
intracellular
intracerebral
intracranial
intractable
intradermal
intradermally
intrahepatic
intraluminal
intramural
intramuscular
intramuscularly
intranasal
intranasally
intransigence
intransigent
intransitive
intra-ocular
intra-orbital
intrapartum
intraperitoneal
intraperitoneally
intraspinal
intrasynovial
intrasynovially
intrathecal
intrathecally
intrathoracic
intra-uterine
intravaginal
intravaginally
intravascular
intravascularly
intravenous
intravenously
intravenous urography
intraventricular
intravesical

intricacies
intricacy
intricate
intrigue
intrigued
intriguing
intrinsic
intrinsically
Intrinsic factor
introduce
introduced
introducer
introducing
introduction
introductory
introitus
introjection
introspection
introspective
introversion
introvert
intrude
intruded
intruding
intrusive
intubate
intubation
intuition
intuitive
intussusception
intussusceptum
intussuscipiens
inunction
inundate
inundated
inundating
inundation
inure
inured
inuring
in utero
invade

invaded
invading
invaginate
invagination
invalid
invalidate
invalidated
invalidating
invalidism
invalidity
invaluable
invaluably
invariable
invariably
invasion
invasiveness
invent
invention
inventor
inventories
inventory
inverse
inversion
invert
invertase
invertebrate
invertor
invest
investigate
investigated
investigating
investigation
investigator
invigorating
invincible
invisible
invisibly
invitation
invite
invited
inviting
in vitro

in vivo
involucrum
involuntarily
involuntary
involute
involuted
involution
involutional
involve
involved
involvement
involving
inward
inwardly
inwards
iodide
iodine
ion
Ionamin®
Ionax Scrub®
ionization
iontophoresis
iota
ipecacuanha
ipratropium
iprindole
ipronazid
ipsilateral
ipsilaterally
ipso facto
Iranian
Iraqui
irascibility
irascible
irascibly
irate
iridectomy
iridescence
iridescent
iridium
iridocyclitis
iridoplegia

iridotomy
iris
irises
Irish
iritis
iron
ironed
ironedetate
ironic
ironical
ironically
ironies
ironing
irony
irradiate
irradiating
irradiation
irrational
irrationally
irreducible
irregular
irregularities
irregularity
irrelevance
irrelevancy
irrelevant
irreparable
irreparably
irreplaceable
irreproachable
irreproachably
irresistible
irresistibly
irrespective
irresponsible
irresponsibly
irrevocable
irrevocably
irrigate
irrigated
irrigating

irrigation
irritability
irritable
irritably
irritant
irritate
irritated
irritating
irritation
irritative
ischaemia
ischaemic
ischial
ischiitis
ischiocavernosus
ischiofemoral
ischiorectal
ischium
Ishihara's colour-
  vision test
island
islander
islet
islets of Langerhans
Ismelin®
isn't
iso-agglutination
isoaminile
isobaric
isocarboxazid
isoconazole
iso-enzyme
isoetharine
isoflurane
Isogel®
iso-immunization
isolate
isolated
isolating
isolation
isolator

isomaltose
isomer
isometheptene
  mucate
isometric
isoniazid
isoprenaline
isosorbide dinitrate
isosorbide
  mononitrate
isotonic
isotopes
isotretinoin
isoxsuprine
ispaghula
Israeli
issue
issued
issuing
isthmus
Italian
italics
itch
itches
itchy
item
itineraries
itinerary
it'll
it's
its
itself
I've
ivermectin
ivory
ivy

Jj

jab
jabbed
jabbing
jackal
jacket
jack-knife
jackpot
Jacksonian epilepsy
Jacuzzi®
jaded
jag
jagged
jagging
jaguar
jail
jailer
Jakob-Creutzfeldt
  disease
jam
jamb
jammed
jamming
janitor
January
jargon
jaundice
jaunt
jaw
jaw-bone
jealous
jealousy
Jectofer®
jejunal
jejunum
jejuostomy
jellies
jelly

jellyfish
Jendrassik's
  manoeuvre
jeopardize
jeopardized
jeopardizing
jeopardy
jerk
jerkily
jerky
jersey
jerseys
jetties
jetty
jewel
jeweler
jeweller
jewellery
jewelry
Jewish
jigsaw
job
Job centre
jockey
jockeyed
jockeying
jocular
jog
jogged
jogging
join
joiner
joint
joist
jollier
jolliest
jollily
jolly
jolt
jostle
jostled
jostling

jotter
joule
journal
journalism
journalist
journey
journeyed
journeying
journeys
jovial
jovially
joyful
joyfully
joyfulness
joyless
joyous
jubilant
jubilation
judge
judged
judgement
judging
judicial
judiciary
judicious
judo
jugular
juice
juicy
ju-jitsu
July
jumble
jumbled
jumbling
jumper
jumpy
junction
junctional
juncture
June
jungle
junior

junk
juries
jurisdiction
jurisprudence
juror
jury
just
justice
justifiable
justifiably
justification
justified
justify
justifying
Juvel®
juvenile
juxta-articular
juxtaglomerular
juxtapose
juxtaposed
juxtaposing
juxtaposition

Kk

Kahn test
kala-azar
kaleidoscope
kallikrein
kallikrein inactivator
Kalspare®
Kalten®
Kamillosan®
kanamycin
kaolin
Kaposi's sarcoma
karate

karaya
kart
karyotype
Kayser-Fleischer ring
kebab
keel
keen
keenness
keep
keeper
keeping
keepsake
Keller's operation
Kell factor
keloid
kelp
kelvin
Kemadrin®
Kenalog®
kennel
kept
keraplasty
keratic
keratin
keratinization
keratinous
keratitis
kerato-acanthoma
keratoconjunctivitis
keratoconjunctivitis
    sicca
keratoderma
keratoderma
    blennorrhagica
keratolysis
keratolytic
keratomalacia
keratoplasty
keratosis
keratosis follicularis
kerb
kerion

Kerley's lines
kernel
kernicterus
Kernig's sign
kerosene
ketamine
ketazolam
ketchup
ketoacidosis
ketoacidotic
ketoconazole
ketogenic
ketonaemia
ketonaemic
ketone
ketonuria
ketonuric
ketoprofen
ketosis
ketosteroid
ketotic
ketotifen
kettle
keyboard
keyed-up
keyhole
keynote
khaki
kick
kick-off
kidnap
kidnapped
kidnapper
kidnapping
kidney
Kielland's forceps
Kienboeck's atrophy
kilocalorie
kilogram
kilogramme
kilometre
kilowatt

Kimmelstiel-Wilson
  disease or syndrome
kinaesthesis
kinaesthetic
kinase
kindergarten
kindliness
kindly
kindness
kindred
kinesia
kinesis
kinetic
kinetically
kingdom
kinin
kininogen
kink
kinsman
kiosk
Kirschner wire
kiss
kisses
kitchen
kitchenette
kitten
Klebsiella
Klebsiella
  pneumoniae
kleptomania
kleptomaniac
Klinefelter syndrome
Kling® bandage
Klippel-Feil disease or
  syndrome
knack
knapsack
knead
knee
kneed
kneeing
kneel

kneeling
knell
knelt
knew
knickers
knick-knack
knife
knifed
knifing
knight
knit
knitted
knitting
knives
knob
knock
knock-kneed
knoll
knot
knotted
knotting
know
knowing
knowingly
knowledge
knowledgeable
knowledgeably
known
knuckle
Kocher's incision
Koch's bacillus
Koebner's
  phenomenon
Köhler's disease
koilonychia
Kolanticon®
Konakion®
Koplik's spots
Korsakoff psychosis
kosher
Kraepelin's
  classification

kraurosis vulvae
Krukenberg tumour
Küntscher nail
kuru
Kussmaul's breathing
  or respiration
Kveim test
kwashiorkor
KY jelly®
kyphoscoliosis
kyphosis
kyphotic

Ll

label
labelled
labelling
labetalol
labia
labial
labia majora
labia minora
labile
lability
labium
laboratories
laboratory
laborious
labour
labourer
labyrinth
labyrinthine
labyrinthitis
lace
laced
lacerate
lacerated

lacerating
laceration
lachesine
lachrymation
lacing
lack
laconic
laconically
lacquer
Lacri-Lube®
lacrimal
lacrimation
lactase
lactate
lactate
  dehydrogenase
  (LDH)
lactation
lactic
lactic acid
lactiferous
Lactobacillus
lactogen
lactose
lactulose
lacuna
lacunae
lacunar
ladder
laden
ladies
lading
ladle
ladled
ladling
lady
ladybird
laevulose
lager
lagoon
laid
lain

laissez faire
laity
lake
lamb
lame
lamella
lamellae
lamellar
lameness
lament
lamentable
lamentation
lamina
laminae
lamina propria
laminated
lamination
laminectomy
lanatoside C
lance
lance-corporal
lanced
Lancefield's groups
lancing
landladies
landlady
landlord
landmark
Landry-Guillain-Barré
  syndrome
landscape
Langhan's giant cell
language
languid
languish
languor
lanky
lanolin
Lanoxin®
lantern
lanugo
lap

laparoscope
laparoscopic
laparoscopically
laparoscopy
laparotomy
lapel
lapped
lapping
lapse
lapsed
lapsing
larceny
larder
Largactil®
large
largesse
larva
larvae
larval
laryngeal
laryngectomy
laryngismus
laryngitis
laryngo-epiglottitis
laryngoscope
laryngoscopic
laryngoscopy
laryngospasm
laryngostenosis
laryngotracheal
laryngotracheitis
laryngotracheo·
  bronchitis
larynx
laser
lash
lashes
Lasikal®
Lasilactone®
Lasix®
Lasix+K®
Lassa fever

Lassar's paste
lassitude
lasso
lassoes
lassos
latamoxef
latch
latches
latchkey
latency
lateness
latent
lateral
laterally
latex
lath
lathe
lather
Latin
latissimus dorsi
latitude
latter
latterly
lattice
laugh
laughable
laughably
laughter
launch
launches
launder
launderette
laundries
laundry
laurel
Laurence-Moon-Biedl
  syndrome
lava
lavage
lavatories
lavatory
lavish

law
lawful
lawfully
lawless
lawlessness
lawn
lawnmower
lawyer
lax
laxative
laxity
Laxoberal®
lay
layby
laybys
layer
layette
laying
laze
lazed
lazier
laziest
lazily
laziness
lazing
lazy
L-dopa
lead
leaden
leader
leading
leaf
leaflet
league
leak
leakage
lean
lean body mass
leaned
leaning
leanness
leant

leap
leaped
leapfrog
leaping
leapt
learn
learned
learner
learning
learnt
lease
leaseback
leased
leasehold
leasing
least
leather
leave
leaves
leaving
leavings
lecherous
lechery
lecithin
lecithinase
lectern
lecture
lectured
lecturer
lecturing
led
Ledercort®
Lederfen®
ledge
ledger
leech
leeches
leek
leeward
leeway
left
legacies

legacy
legal
legalities
legality
legally
legend
legendary
legibility
legible
legibly
legion
legionary
Legionella
legionnaires' disease
legislate
legislated
legislating
legislation
legislative
legislator
legislature
legitimacy
legitimate
legume
leguminous
leiomyofibroma
leiomyoma
Leishman-Donovan
  bodies
Leishmania
leishmaniacides
Leishmania donovani
leishmaniasis
leisure
lemniscus
lemon
lemonade
lend
lending
length
lengthen
lengthily

lengthways
lengthy
leniency
lenient
lens
lenses
lent
Lent
Lentard MC®
lente
lenticular
lentigines
lentigo
Lentizol®
leopard
leper
lepra
leprid
lepride
leproma
lepromata
lepromatous
leprosy
leprous
Leptospira
Leptospira
  icterohaemorrhagiae
leptospirosis
lesbian
lesbianism
lesion
less
lessen
lesser
lesson
lest
let
lethal
lethargic
lethargically
lethargy
letter

Letterer-Siwe disease
letting
lettuce
leucine
leucoblast
leucoblastosis
leucocyte
leucocytic
leucocytosis
leucocytotic
leucodystrophy
leuconychia
leucopenia
leucopenic
leucoplakia
leucopoiesis
leucopoietic
leucorrhoea
leucorrhoeal
leucotomy
leucovorin
leukaemia
leukaemic
leukodystrophy
leukoplakia
levamisole
levator
levator ani
level
levelled
levelling
lever
levied
levies
Levin tube
levity
levodopa
levonorgestrel
levorphanol
levy
levying
lewd

lewdness
lexicographer
lexicography
Leydig
liabilities
liability
liable
liaise
liaised
liaising
liaison
liar
libel
libelled
libelling
libellous
liberal
liberality
liberally
liberation
liberties
liberty
libidinous
libido
librarian
libraries
library
Librium®
lice
licence
license
licensed
licensee
licensing
licentious
lichen
lichenification
lichenoid
lichen planus
lichen sclerosus et
  atrophicus
lick

lidoflazine
lie
lied
lienculus
lienorenal
lieu
lieutenant
life
lifeguard
lifeless
life-like
ligament
ligamentous
ligate
ligation
ligature
light
lighted
lighten
lighter
lighthouse
lighting
lightning
lightning pains
lignocaine
likable
like
likeable
liked
likelihood
likely
likeness
likewise
liking
lilies
lily
limb
limber
limbic
limbus
limelight
liminal

limit
limitation
limited
limiting
limousine
limpid
linchpin
lincomycin
linctus
lindane
line
linea
linea alba
linea aspera
lineage
lineal
lineally
lineament
linear
lined
linen
lingerie
lingual
linguist
linguistic
linguistically
linguistics
lingula
liniment
lining
linolenic acid
linoleum
linseed
lint
lintel
Lioresal®
liothyronine
lipaemia
lipaemic
lipase
lipid
lipidaemia

lipodystrophy
lipogenesis
lipoid
lipoidoses
lipoidosis
lipolysis
lipolytic
lipoma
lipomata
lipomatous
lipoprotein
lipotrophic
lipstick
liquefaction
liquefied
liquefy
liquefying
liqueur
liquid
liquidate
liquidated
liquidating
liquidation
liquidator
liquidity
liquid paraffin
Liquifilm®
liquor
liquorice
lisinopril
lissom
lissome
listen
listened
listener
listening
Listeria
Listeria
  monocytogenes
listless
lit
literacy

literal
literally
literary
literate
literature
lithe
lithiasis
lithium
lithotomy
lithotripsy
lithotriptor
litmus
litre
litter
little
Little's area
live
lived
livedo
livelier
liveliest
livelihood
liveliness
livelong
lively
liver
lives
living
living-room
loaf
loafed
loafing
Loa loa
loam
loan
loath
loathe
loathed
loathing
loaves
lobar
lobbies

lobby
lobe
lobectomy
lobotomy
lobster
lobular
lobulated
lobule
local
locale
locality
localization
localize
localized
localizing
locate
located
locating
location
lochia
lochial
locker
lockjaw
lock-out
Locoid®
locomotion
locomotor
Locorten-Vioform®
loculated
locum
locums
locum tenens
locus
locust
lodge
lodged
lodger
lodging
Loestrin 20®
Loestrin 30®
Loewenstein-Jensen
  culture medium

lofepramine
loftily
loftiness
lofty
log
logbook
logged
loggerheads
logging
logic
logical
logically
logo
logorrhoea
logos
Logynon®
Logynon ED®
loiasis
loin
loincloth
loiter
Lomotil®
lomustine
lone
loneliness
lonely
lonesome
long
longevity
longing
longissimus muscle
longitude
lookout
loop
loophole
loose
loosen
loperamide
Lopid®
loprazolam
lop-sided
loquacious

lorazepam
lordly
lordosis
lordship
lore
Lorexane®
lormetazepam
lorries
lorry
lose
loser
losing
loss
losses
lost
loth
lotion
lotio rubra
lotteries
lottery
loud
loudness
loudspeaker
Louis (Angle of)
lounge
lounged
lounging
lour
louse
lovable
lovelier
loveliest
loveliness
lovely
lower
lowered
lowering
lowland
lowliness
lowly
lowness
loyal

loyally
loyalty
lozenge
lubb
lubb-dupp
lubricant
lubricate
lubricated
lubricating
lubrication
lucid
lucidity
luckier
luckiest
luckily
lucky
lucrative
ludicrous
Ludiomil®
Ludwig's angina
Luer's syringe
luetic
luetin
luggage
Lugol's solution
lugubrious
lukewarm
lumbago
lumbar
lumbarization
lumbar puncture
lumber
lumbosacral
lumbrical
lumen
lumina
luminal
Luminal®
luminosity
luminous
lumpectomy
lunacy

lunate
lunatic
lunch
luncheon
lunches
lung
lunge
lunged
lunging
lupoid
lupus
lupus erythematosus
lupus pernio
lurk
luscious
lustre
lustrous
luteal
luteinization
luteinizing hormone
luteum
luxuriant
luxuriate
luxuriated
luxuriating
luxuries
luxurious
luxury
lying
lymecycline
Lyme disease
lymph
lymphadenitis
lymphadenopathy
lymphangiectasia
lymphangiectasis
lymphangiogram
lymphangiography
lymphangioma
lymphangiomata
lymphangitis
lymphatic

lymph gland
lymphoblast
lymphoblastic
lymphoblastoma
lymphocyte
lymphocytic
lymphocytosis
lymphoedema
lymphogram
lymphogranuloma
  inguinale
lymphogranuloma
  venereum
lymphography
lymphoid
lymphoma
lymphomata
lymphomatosis
lymphomatous
lymphoreticular
lymphosarcoma
lymphosarcomata
lymphosarcomatous
lynch
lynoestrenol
lypressin
lyric
lyrical
lyrically
lysergic acid
  diethylamide (LSD)
lysergide
lysin
lysine
lysis
lysogeny
lysosome
lysozyme

Mm

Maalox®
macabre
macerated
maceration
MacEwen's operation
  or osteotomy
machine
machinery
machinist
mackintosh
mackintoshes
macrocyte
macrocytic
macrocytosis
macroeconomics
macroglobulin
macroglobulinaemia
macroglossia
macrognathia
macrogol
macrophages
macroscopic
macula
macular
macule
maculopapular
mad
madam
madden
madder
maddest
made
madman
madmen
madness
Madopar®
mafenide
magaldrate

Mm

magazine
maggot
maggoty
magic
magical
magically
magician
magisterial
magistrate
magnanimity
magnanimous
Magnapen®
magnate
magnesia
magnesium
magnet
magnetic
magnetically
magnetism
magnetize
magnetized
magnetizing
magnification
magnificence
magnificent
magnified
magnify
magnifying
magnitude
magnum
maim
mainframe
mainland
mainly
mainstay
maintain
maintained
maintaining
maintenance
maize
major
majorities

majority
make
maker
makeshift
make-up
making
mal
malabsorption
malacia
maladies
maladjusted
maladjustment
malady
malaise
malalignment
malar
malaria
malarial
malathion
male
malevolent
malformation
malformed
malice
malicious
malign
malignancy
malignant
malingerer
malingering
malleable
malleolar
malleoli
malleolus
malleus
Mallory-Weiss
  syndrome
malnutrition
malocclusion
malodorous
Maloprim®
Malpighian corpuscle

malposition
malpractice
malpresentation
maltase
maltose
maltreat
maltreatment
malunion
mama
mamma
mammal
mammary
mammillary bodies
mammogram
mammographic
mammographically
mammography
mammoplasty
mammoth
man
manage
manageable
managed
management
manager
manageress
managing
Manchester operation
mandate
mandatory
mandible
mandibular
mange
mangy
manhandle
manhandled
manhandling
manhood
mania
maniac
manic
manic-depressive

manicure
manicurist
manifest
manifestation
manifesto
manifestoes
manifestos
manipulate
manipulated
manipulating
manipulation
manned
manner
mannerism
manning
mannish
mannitol
manoeuvre
manometer
manometric
manpower
manslaughter
mantelpiece
mantle
Mantoux reaction or test
manual
manually
manubrium
manufacture
manufactured
manufacturer
manufacturing
manuscript
many
map
maple syrup urine disease
mapped
mapping
maprotiline
mar

marasmic
marasmus
marble
marble bones
Marcain®
march
March
marches
Marevan®
Marfan's syndrome
margarine
margin
marginal
marginally
marijuana
marine
marital
maritime
marjoram
mark
marked
marker
market
marketed
marketing
marred
marriage
married
marring
marrow
marry
marrying
marsh
marshal
marshalled
marshalling
Marshall-Marchetti-Krantz operation
marshes
marshy
marsupial
marsupialization

martyr
marvel
marvelled
marvelling
marvellous
Marvelon®
mascot
masculine
masculinity
masculinization
masculinize
masked
masochism
masochist
masochistic
masochistically
mason
masonic
mass
massage
massaged
massaging
Masse ®
masses
masseter
masseur
masseuse
massive
mastalgia
mastectomy
master
masterly
mastery
masticate
masticated
masticating
mastication
mastitis
mastocyte
mastocytosis
mastoid
mastoidectomy

Mm

mastoiditis
masturbate
masturbated
masturbating
masturbation
mat
match
matchbox
matchboxes
matches
matchless
mate
mated
materia
material
materialism
materialize
materialized
materializing
materially
maternal
maternally
maternity
mathematical
mathematically
mathematician
mathematics
mating
matrices
matriculate
matriculated
matriculating
matriculation
matrimonial
matrimony
matrix
matron
matt
matte
matted
matter
matter-of-fact

matting
mattress
mattresses
maturation
mature
matured
maturing
maturity
Maxepa®
Maxidex®
maxilla
maxillary
maxillofacial
maxim
maxima
maximal
maximum
Maxitrol®
Maxolon®
may
May
maybe
Mayo's operation
mazindol
McArdle's disease
McBurney's point
McMurray's
  osteotomy
McNaghten's Rules
meagre
meagrely
meal
mean
meaning
meaningless
meanness
meant
meanwhile
measles
measly
measure
measured

measurement
measuring
meatal
meatotomy
meatus
mebendazole
mebeverine
mebhydrolin
mechanic
mechanical
mechanically
mechanics
mechanism
mechanize
mechanized
mechanizing
mecillinam
Meckel's diverticulum
meclozine
meconium
meconium ileus
medal
medallion
medallist
medazepam
meddle
meddled
meddling
media
mediaeval
medial
medially
median
mediastinal
mediastinitis
mediastinoscopy
mediastinum
mediate
mediated
mediating
mediation
mediator

medical
medically
medicament
medicamentosa
medicamentosus
medicated
medication
medicinal
medicine
medicochirurgical
medicolegal
medieval
Medihaler®
mediocre
mediocrity
mediolateral
meditate
meditated
meditating
meditation
Mediterranean
medium
mediums
medius
Medrone®
medroxyprogesterone
medulla
medulla oblongata
medullary
medulloblastoma
meet
meeting
mefenamic
mefruside
megabyte
megacolon
megakaryocyte
megaloblast
megaloblastic
megalomania
megaphone
megaton

megestrol
meibomian cyst
meibomian gland
Meigs syndrome
meiosis
Meissner's corpuscle
melaena
melancholia
melancholic
melancholy
melanin
melanocyte
melanoma
melanomata
melanomatous
melanosis
melanotic
melatonin
melitensis
Melleril®
melodies
melody
melphalan
melt
member
membership
membrane
membranous
memo
memoir
memorable
memorably
memoranda
memorandum
memorandums
memories
memorize
memorized
memorizing
memory
memos
men

menadiol
menarche
Mendelian theory
Ménière's disease
meningeal
meninges
meningioma
meningiomatous
meningism
meningitis
meningocele
meningococcaemia
meningococcal
meningococcus
meningo-encephalitis
meningo-encephalo·
  myelitis
meningomyelocele
meniscectomy
menisci
meniscus
menopausal
menopause
Menophase®
menorrhagia
menotrophin
menses
menstrual
menstruate
menstruated
menstruating
menstruation
mental
mentalities
mentality
mentally
menthol
mention
mentioned
mentioning
mento-anterior
mentoposterior

Mm

mentor
menu
menus
mepacrine
mepenzolate
meprobamate
meptazinol
mequitazine
Merbentyl®
mercantile
mercaptopurine
Mercilon®
mercurial
mercuric
mercurochrome
mercury
mercy
mere
merely
merge
merged
merger
merging
merit
merited
meriting
merozoite
merrier
merriest
merrily
merry
mersalyl
mesalazine
mescaline
mesencephalon
mesenchymal
mesenchyme
mesenteric
mesentery
mesh
meshes
mesmerism

mesmerize
mesmerized
mesmerizing
mesna
meso-
mesoderm
mesodermal
mesomorph
mesomorphic
mesothelioma
mess
message
messenger
messes
Messrs
mesterolone
Mestinon®
met
metabolic
metabolically
metabolism
metabolite
metabolize
metacarpal
metacarpophalangeal
metacarpus
metal
metallic
metallurgical
metallurgy
metamorphic
metamorphopsia
metamorphoses
metamorphosis
metamyelocyte
metaphase
metaphor
metaphorical
metaphorically
metaphyseal
metaphysis
metaplasia

metaplastic
metaraminol
metastases
metastasis
metastasize
metastatic
metatarsal
metatarsalgia
metatarsophalangeal
metatarsus
meted out
meteor
meteoric
meteorite
meteorological
meteorologically
meteorologist
meteorology
mete out
meter
metformin
methadone
methaemalbumin
methaemoglobin
methaemoglobin·
  aemia
methane
methicillin
methionine
methionyl
methixene
methocarbamol
method
methodical
methodically
methohexitone
methotrexate
methotrimeprazine
methoxamine
methoxsalen
methyclothiazide
methylated

methylated spirit
methylcellulose
methylcysteine
methyldopa
methyldopate
methylene blue
methylphenobarbitone
methylprednisolone
methyl salicylate
methyltestosterone
methyprylone
methysergide
meticulous
meting out
metipranolol
metirosine
metoclopramide
metolazone
metoprolol
Metosyn®
metre
metric
metrical
metricate
metricated
metricating
metrication
metriphonate
metronidazole
metropathia
  haemorrhagica
metropolitan
metrorrhagia
metyrapone
mexiletine
mezlocillin
mianserin
mice
micelle
Micolette®
miconazole
Micralax®

micro-aerophilic
micro-angiopathy
microbe
microbial
microbiologist
microbiology
microcephalic
microcephaly
microchip
microcirculation
microclimate
Micrococcus
microcomputer
microcosm
microcyte
microcytic
microcytosis
microeconomics
microenvironment
microfiche
microfilaria
microfilm
micrognathia
microgram
Microgynon 30®
micron
Micronor®
microphone
Micropore®
microprocessor
microscope
microscopic
microscopy
microsecond
Microsporum
microsurgery
microsurgical
Microval®
microwave
Mictral®
micturate
Micturin®

micturition
midazolam
mid-brain
mid-cycle
midday
middle
middle-aged
middle-class
midget
mid-gut
midnight
midriff
midst
midway
midwife
midwifery
midwives
might
mightier
mightiest
mightily
mighty
migraine
migrainous
Migraleve®
migratory
Migravess®
Migril®
mike
milage
mild
mildew
mile
mileage
milestone
miliaria
miliary
miliary tuberculosis
milieu
military
milium
millaria

Mm

millennia
millennium
miller
millicurie
milli-equivalent
milligram
milligramme
millilitre
millimetre
million
millionaire
millivolt
Milton®
Milwaukee brace
mimic
mimicked
mimicking
mimicry
mince
minced
mincemeat
mincer
mincing
mind
mindful
mindless
mine
mineral
mineralocorticoid
mineralogist
mineralogy
mingle
mingled
mingling
mini
miniature
minibus
minibuses
minicomputer
Minihep®
Min-i-Jet®
Minilyn®

minim
minima
minimal
minimize
minimized
minimizing
Minims®
minimum
minis
minister
ministerial
ministerially
ministries
ministry
minium
Minocin®
minocycline
minor
minorities
minority
Minovlar®
minoxidil
mint
Mintezol®
Minulet®
minus
minute
minutes
miosis
miotic
miracle
miraculous
mire
mirror
mirth
misadventure
misanthrope
misbehave
misbehaved
misbehaving
misbehaviour
miscarriage

miscarried
miscarry
miscarrying
miscellaneous
miscellanies
miscellany
mischance
mischief
mischievous
miscible
misconception
misconduct
misdeed
misdemeanour
miser
miserable
miserably
misfit
misfortune
misgiving
misguided
mishap
mislaid
mislay
mislaying
mislead
misleading
misled
misnomer
misoprostol
misprint
miss
missed
missed abortion
misses
misshapen
missing
mission
missive
misspell
misspelled
misspelling

misspelt
misspent
mistake
mistaken
mistaking
mistook
mistrust
misty
misunderstand
misunderstanding
misunderstood
misuse
mitigating
mitobronitol
mitochondria
mitochondrion
mitomycin
mitosis
mitotic
mitozantrone
mitral
mitral incompetence
mitral stenosis .
mitral valvotomy or
  valvulotomy
mittelschmerz
mix
mixed
mixer
mixes
Mixtard 30/70®
mixture
mnemonic
moan
mob
mobbed
mobbing
mobile
mobility
mobilization
mobilize
mobilized

mobilizing
mock
mockery
mocking
mode
Modecate®
model
modelled
modelling
modem
moderate
moderation
modern
modernity
modernization
modernize
modernized
modernizing
modest
modesty
modicum
modification
modified
modify
modifying
Moditen®
Moducren®
modulation
Moduretic®
Mogadon®
moist
moisten
moistened
moistening
moisture
moisturize
moisturized
moisturizing
molar
molarity
mole
molecular

molecule
molest
Molipaxin®
mollusc
molluscum
molluscum
  contagiosum
molten
moment
momentarily
momentary
momentous
momentum
monarthritis
monarticular
Mönckeberg's
  sclerosis
Monday
monetarism
monetary
money
mongol
mongolism
mongoloid
mongrel
Monilia
monilial
moniliasis
Monistat®
monitor
monitoring
monoamine-oxidase
monocular
monocyte
monocytic
monogamy
monogram
monolayer
monomer
mononeuritis
mononeuritis multiplex
mononuclear

Mm

mononucleosis
Monophane®
monoplegia
monopolies
monopolize
monopolized
monopolizing
monopoly
monosaccharide
monosodium
  glutamate
monosulfiram
monosyllabic
monosynaptic
Monotard®
monotonous
monotony
monovalent
monozygotic
Monphytol®
mons
monster
monstrosities
monstrosity
monstrous
month
monthlies
monthly
monument
monumental
moonbeam
moonlight
moot point
mope
moped
moping
moral
morale
morality
morally
morass
morasses

morbid
morbidity
morbilliform
more
moreover
morgue
moribund
morn
morning
moron
moronic
Moro reflex
morose
morphia
morphine
morphoea
morphogenesis
morphological
morphologically
morphology
morrow
morse
morsel
mortal
mortality
mortally
mortgage
mortgaged
mortgaging
mortice
mortified
mortify
mortifying
mortise
Morton's
  metatarsalgia
mortuaries
mortuary
morula
mosaic
mosaicism
Moslem

mosquito
mosquitoes
mosquitos
moss
mosses
mossy
most
mote
moth
mothball
moth-eaten
mother
motherhood
mother-in-law
motherly
mothers-in-law
motile
motility
motion
motionless
Motipress®
Motival®
motivate
motivated
motivating
motive
motor
motor-bike
motorcycle
motorist
motorize
motorized
motorizing
motorway
mottled
motto
mottoes
mould
moulder
mouldy
moult
mound

mount
mountain
mountaineer
mourn
mourner
mourning
mouse
mousse
moustache
mousy
mouth
mouthful
mouthfuls
mouth-wash
movable
move
moveable
moved
movement
movie
moving
mower
Mr
Mrs
Ms
MST Continus®
Mucaine®
much
mucilaginous
mucin
mucinolysis
mucinolytic
mucinous
muck
mucocele
mucocutaneous
mucoid
mucolytic
mucopolysaccharide
mucopolysacchar·
  idoses

mucopolysacchar·
  idosis
mucopurulent
mucopus
mucosa
mucosae
mucosal
mucous
mucoviscidosis
mucus
muddle
muddled
muddling
muddy
mudguard
mule
multi-coloured
multifarious
multigravida
multigravidae
multilobular
multilocular
multimillionaire
multinational
multinodular
multinuclear
multinucleate
multipara
multiparae
multiparous
multiple
multiple sclerosis
  (MS)
multiplex
multiplication
multiplicity
multiplied
multiply
multiplying
multitude
multitudinous

multivitamin
mummies
mummification
mummy
mumps
munch
Munchausen
  syndrome
municipal
municipalities
municipality
mupirocin
mural
murder
murderer
murderous
murine
murky
murmur
murmured
murmuring
Murphy's sign
muscle
muscle relaxant
muscular
muscular dystrophies
muscular dystrophy
muscularis mucosae
muscularity
musculature
musculocutaneous
musculoskeletal
museum
mushroom
mushy
music
musical
musically
musician
Muslim
muslin

musquash
mussel
must
mustard
mustine
musty
mutagen
mutagenesis
mutagenic
mutant
mutase
mutation
mute
muted
mutilate
mutilated
mutilating
mutilation
mutism
mutton
mutual
mutually
myalgia
myalgic
myalgic
  encephalomyelitis
myasthenia
myasthenia gravis
myasthenic
myatonia
myatonia congenita
mycelial
mycelium
mycetoma
mycetome
Mycobacteriaceae
Mycobacterium
Mycobacterium leprae
Mycobacterium
  tuberculosis
mycological
mycologist

mycology
Mycoplasma
Mycoplasma
  pneumoniae
mycosis
mycosis fungoides
Mycota®
mycotic
mydriasis
mydriatic
Mydrilate®
myelin
myelinated
myelination
myelitis
myeloblast
myeloblastic
myelocele
myelocyte
myelocytic
myelofibrosis
myelogenous
myelogram
myelographic
myelography
myeloid
myeloma
myelomata
myelomatosis
myelomatous
myelomeningocele
myelopathy
myeloradiculography
myelosclerosis
myocardial
myocardial infarction
myocarditis
myocardium
myoclonic
myoclonus
Myocrisin®
Myodil®

myofibril
myofibrosis
myogenic
myoglobin
myoma
myomata
myomatous
myomectomy
myometrial
myometrium
myoneural
myopathic
myopathy
myope
myopia
myopic
myopically
myosarcoma
myosin
myositis
myotomy
myotonia
myotonia congenita
myotonic
myriad
myringitis
myringoplasty
myringotomy
Mysoline®
Mysteclin®
mysteries
mysterious
mystery
mystified
mystify
mystifying
myth
mythical
mythically
mythological
mythology
myxoedema

myxoedematous
myxoma
myxomata
myxomatosis
myxomatous
myxovirus

Nn

nabilone
nabothian follicle
nabumetone
nadolol
naevi
naevoid
naevus
naftidrofuryl
  oxalate
nail
nailing
naive
naiveté
naked
nalbuphine
nalidixic acid
Nalorex®
naloxone
naltrezone
name
named
namely
naming
nandrolone
  decanoate
nandrolone
  phenylpropionate
nannies
nanny
nanogram

nanometre
nanosecond
nape
napkin
napkin dermatitis
nappies
nappy
nappy rash
Naprosyn®
naproxen
Narcan®
narcissi
narcissism
narcissistic
narcissus
narcolepsy
narcoleptic
narcosis
narcotic
Nardil®
nares
naris
narrate
narrated
narrating
narration
narrative
narrator
narrow
nasal
Naseptin®
nasogastric
nasolacrimal
nasopharyngeal
nasopharynx
nastily
nastiness
nasturtium
nasty
natal
natamycin
nation

national
nationalism
nationalities
nationality
nationalization
nationalize
nationalized
nationalizing
nationally
native
nativity
Natrilix®
natriuresis
natural
naturalist
naturalize
naturalized
naturalizing
naturally
nature
naturopathic
naturopathy
naughtily
naughtiness
naughty
nausea
nauseate
nauseated
nauseating
nauseous
nautical
naval
navel
navicular
Navidrex®
Navidrex-K®
navies
navigable
navigate
navigated
navigating
navigation

Nn

navigator
navy
Nebuhaler®
Nebules®
nebulization
nebulize
nebulizer
nebulous
Necator
Necator
 americanus
necatoriasis
necessarily
necessary
necessitate
necessitated
necessitating
necessities
necessity
necklace
necrobiosis
necrobiosis
 lipoidica
 diabeticorum
necropolis
necropolises
necropsy
necrosis
necrotic
necrotizing
 enterocolitis
 (NEC)
nedocromil
née
needful
needle
needless
needy
nefarious
nefopam
negate
negated

negating
negative
negativism
neglect
neglectful
negligence
negligent
negligible
negligibly
negotiable
negotiate
negotiated
negotiating
negotiation
negotiator
Negram®
Negress
Negro
Negroes
neighbour
neighbourhood
neighbouring
Neisseria
Neisseria
 gonorrhoeae
Neisseria
 meningitidis
neither
nematode
Neocon-1/35®
Neo-Cortef®
Neo-Cytamen®
Neogest®
neologism
Neo-Medrone®
neomycin
Neo-NaClex®
Neo-NaClex-K®
neonatal
neonate
neonatology
neonatorum

neon lighting
neoplasia
neoplasm
neoplastic
Neosporin®
neostigmine
Nepenthe®
nephew
nephrectomy
Nephril®
nephritic
nephritis
nephroblastoma
nephrocalcinosis
nephrogenic
nephrolithiasis
nephrolithotomy
nephrology
nephroma
nephron
nephropathic
nephropathy
nephropexy
nephroptosis
nephrosis
nephrostomy
nephrotic
nephrotic
 syndrome
nephrotomy
nephrotoxic
nephrotoxin
Nerisone®
nerve
nervous
nervousness
net
netball
nether
netilmicin
nett
netted

netting
nettle
network
Neulactil®
neural
neuralgia
neuralgic
neural tube defect
neurasthenia
neurasthenic
neurectomy
neurilemma
neurilemmoma
neuritic
neuritis
neuro-anatomy
neuroblast
neuroblastoma
neurochemistry
neurodermatitis
neuro-endocrine
neurofibril
neurofibrillar
neurofibroma
neurofibromata
neurofibromatosis
neurofibromatous
neurogenic
neuroglia
neuroglial
neuroleptic
neurological
neurologist
neurology
neuroma
neuromuscular
neuron
neuronal
neurone
neuropathic
neuropathological
neuropathology

neuropathy
neuropeptide
neuropharma·
  cological
neuropharmacology
neurophysiologist
neurophysiology
neuropsychiatric
neuropsychiatry
neuroradiologist
neuroradiology
neuroses
neurosis
neurosurgeon
neurosurgery
neurosurgical
neurosyphilis
neurotic
neuroticism
neurotomy
neurotoxic
neurotoxin
neurotropic
neurovascular
neuter
neutral
neutrality
neutralization
neutralize
neutralized
neutralizing
neutrally
neutron
neutropenia
neutropenic
neutrophil
neutrophilia
never
nevertheless
newly
newness
newsagent

newspaper
newt
nibble
nibbled
nibbling
nicardipine
nice
niceties
nicety
niche
nickel
nickname
niclosamide
nicofuranose
nicotinamide
nicotinate
nicotine
nicotinic
nicotinic acid
nicotinyl
nicoumalone
nidus
niece
Niemann-Pick disease
nifedipine
nigh
nightdress
nightfall
nightingale
nightmare
night-terror
nihilistic
nikethamide
nimble
nimbly
nimodipine
nimorazole
Nimotop®
nine
nineteen
nineteenth
ninetieth

Nn

ninety
ninth
nip
nipped
nipping
nipple
niridazole
Nissl degeneration
nitrate
nitrazepam
nitric
nitrite
nitrofurantoin
nitrofurazone
nitrogen
nitrogenous
nitroglycerine
Nitrolingual®
nitrophenol
nitroprusside
nitrous
nitrous oxide
Nivaquine®
nizatidine
Nizoral®
no
nobility
noble
nobly
nobody
nocturia
nocturnal
nocturnally
nodal
node
nodular
nodule
noes
noise
noisily
noisy
nomenclature

nominal
nominally
nominate
nominated
nominating
nomination
nominee
nomogram
nonagenarian
non-articular
nonchalance
nonchalant
non-committal
non compos mentis
nonconformist
non-consummation
non-depolarizing
nondescript
non-disjunction
none
nonentities
nonentity
non-Hodgkin's
  lymphoma
non-invasive
non-motile
nonoxinol
nonplussed
nonsense
nonsensical
nonsensically
non sequitur
non-specific urethritis
non-steroidal anti-
  inflammatory drugs
  (NSAID)
non-union
non-viable
non-voting
Noonan syndrome
no-one
noradrenaline

norepinephrine
norethisterone
Norflex®
Norgeston®
norgestrel
Noriday®
Norimin®
Norinyl-1®
Noristerat®
Normacol®
normal
normally
normoblast
normoblastic
normochromic
normocyte
normocytic
normoglycaemia
normoglycaemic
normotension
normotensive
north
northerly
northern
nortriptyline
Norwegian
noscapine
nosey
nosological
nosology
nostalgia
nostalgic
nostalgically
nostril
nosy
notably
notation
notch
notches
note
noted
noteworthy

nothing
notice
noticeable
noticeably
noticed
noticing
notifiable
notification
notified
notify
notifying
noting
notion
notochord
notoriety
notorious
notwithstanding
nougat
nought
noun
nourish
nourishment
novel
novelist
novelties
novelty
November
novice
NovoPen®
nowadays
nowhere
noxious
Noxyflex®
noxythiolin
nozzle
nuance
nuchal
nuclear
nuclear magnetic
  resonance (NMR)

nucleated
nuclei
nucleide
nucleolar
nucleolus
nucleoprotein
nucleotides
nucleus
nudge
nudged
nudging
nudist
nudity
Nuelin®
nuisance
null
nullified
nullify
nullifying
nullipara
nulliparity
nulliparous
numb
number
numbered
numbering
numeracy
numeral
numerate
numerical
numerically
numerous
nummular
nun
nuptial
nurse
nursed
nurseries
nursery
nursing

nurture
nurtured
nurturing
Nu-Seals Aspirin
nutrient
nutriment
nutrition
nutritional
nutritionist
nutritious
nutshell
nux vomica
nylon
nymphomania
nymphomaniac
Nystaform®
Nystaform-HC®
nystagmograph
nystagmography
nystagmus
nystatin

Oo

oases
oasis
oat cell carcinoma
oath
oaths
oats
obedience
obedient
obeisance
obese
obesity
obey
obfuscation
obituaries
obituary

object
objection
objectionable
objectionably
objective
obligate
obligation
obligatorily
obligatory
oblige
obliged
obliging
oblique
obliquity
obliquus
obliterate
obliterated
obliterating
oblitertation
oblivion
oblivious
oblong
obnoxious
obscene
obscenities
obscenity
obscure
obscurity
obsequious
observance
observant
observation
observatories
observatory
observe
observed
observer
observing
obsess
obsession
obsessional neurosis
obsessive

obsessive-compulsive
obsolescence
obsolescent
obsolete
obsructive
obstacle
obstetrical
obstetrician
obstetrics
obstinacy
obstinate
obstreperous
obstruct
obstruction
obstructive
obtain
obtainable
obtrusive
obturator
obtuse
obvious
obviously
occasion
occasional
occasionally
occipital
occipitoanterior
occipitofrontalis
occipitoparietal
occipitoposterior
occiput
occlude
occlusion
occlusive
occult
occult blood
occupancy
occupant
occupation
occupational disease
occupied
occupier

occupy
occupying
occur
occurred
occurrence
occurring
ocean
o'clock
octagonal
octagonally
October
octogenarian
octopus
octopuses
octoxinol
ocular
oculist
oculogyric
oculomotor
Ocusert Pilo®
Ocusol®
oddities
oddity
oddment
odious
odontoid
odour
odourless
oedema
oedematous
Oedipus complex
oesophageal
oesophagectomy
oesophagitis
oesophagoscope
oesophagoscopic
oesophagoscopy
oesophagostomy
oesophagotomy
oesophagus
oestone
oestradiol

oestriol
oestrogen
oestrogenic
oestrus
offal
off-chance
offence
offend
offender
offensive
offer
offhand
office
officer
official
officially
officiate
officiated
officiating
officious
offing
off-licence
offset
offsetting
offshoot
offside
offspring
often
Oilatum®
oilfield
oilrig
oily
ointment
old-fashioned
olecranon
olecranon bursitis
olfaction
olfactory
oligaemia
oligaemic
oligohydramnios
oligomenorrhoea

oligospermia
oliguria
oliguric
olive
omega
omega-3 marine
  triglyceride
omelet
omelette
omen
omental
omentum
ominous
omission
omit
omitted
omitting
omnibus
omnibuses
omnipotent
omniscient
omnivorous
Omnopon®
omohyoid
omphalocele
once
Onchocerca
Onchocerca volvulus
onchocerciasis
oncogene
oncogenic
oncological
oncologically
oncology
oncolysis
oncolytic
oncoming
onerous
oneself
ongoing
onion
onlooker

onslaught
onus
onwards
onychogryphosis
onycholysis
onychomycosis
onyx
oocyte
oogenesis
oogenetic
oophorectomy
ooze
oozed
oozing
opacification
opacity
opal
opaque
open
open-angle glaucome
opened
opening
operability
operable
operant conditioning
operate
operated
operating
operation
operative
operator
Ophthaine®
ophthalmia
ophthalmia
  neonatorum
ophthalmic
ophthalmological
ophthalmologically
ophthalmologist
ophthalmology
ophthalmoplegia
ophthalmoplegic

ophthalmoscope
ophthalmoscopic
ophthalmoscopy
opiate
Opilon®
opinion
opinionated
opioid
opium
opponens
opponens digiti minimi
opponens pollicis
opponent
opportune
opportunism
opportunist
opportunistic infection
opportunities
opportunity
oppose
opposed
opposing
opposite
opposition
oppression
oppressive
opsonin
optic
optical
optician
Opticrom®
optics
optimal
Optimax®
Optimine®
optimism
optimist
optimistic
optimistically
optimum
option
optional

optionally
optometrist
optometry
opulence
opulent
Opulets®
Orabase®
oral
oral contraceptive
Oraldene®
oral hypoglycaemic
orally
orange
orang-utan
Orap®
oration
orator
orbicular
orbicularis oculi
orbit
orbital
orchard
orchestra
orchid
orchidectomy
orchidopexy
orchitis
orciprenaline
ordain
ordeal
order
orderlies
orderly
ordinal
ordinance
ordinarily
ordinary
ordination
orf
organ
organic
organically

organification
organism
organization
organize
organized
organizing
organ of Corti
organophosphorus
orgasm
orgies
orgy
orient
oriental
orientation
orienteering
orifice
origin
original
originally
originate
originated
originating
ornament
ornate
ornithine
ornithological
ornithologist
ornithology
ornithosis
oro-antral
orogenital
oropharyngeal
oropharynx
orphan
orphanage
orphenadrine
Ortho-Creme®
Ortho Dienoestrol®
orthodontic
orthodox
orthodox sleep
orthodoxy

Orthoforms®
orthography
Ortho-Gynest®
Ortho-Gynol®
Ortho-Novin 1/50®
orthopaedic
orthopnoea
orthopnoeic
orthoptic
orthoptics
orthostatic
Ortolani's sign
Orudis®
Oruvail®
os
oscillate
oscillated
oscillating
oscillation
oscilloscope
Osgood-Schlatter's
   disease
Osler's nodes
osmolality
osmolar
osmolarity
osmole
osmoreceptor
osmoregulatory
osmosis
osmotic
osmotic pressure
osseous
ossicle
ossification
ossify
Ossopan®
osteitis
ostensible
ostensibly
ostentation
ostentatious

osteoarthritic
osteoarthritis
osteo-arthropathy
osteoarthrosis
osteoblast
osteoblastic
osteochondritis
osteochondroma
osteoclast
osteoclastic
osteoclastoma
osteocyte
osteodystrophy
osteogenesis
   imperfecta
osteogenic
osteolytic
osteoma
osteomalacia
osteomyelitis
osteopath
osteopathic
osteopathy
osteopetrosis
osteophyte
osteophytic
osteophytosis
osteoporosis
osteoporotic
osteosarcoma
osteosarcomata
osteosarcomatous
osteotomy
ostia
ostial
ostium
ostomy seal
ostracism
ostracize
ostracized
ostracizing
ostrich

ostriches
otalgia
other
otitis
otitis externa
otitis media
otolaryngology
otolith
otologist
otology
otorhinolaryngology
otorrhoea
otosclerosis
otosclerotic
otoscope
otoscopic
otoscopy
Otosporin®
ototoxic
Otrivine®
Otrivine-Antistin®
ought
ounce
ourselves
oust
outboard
outbreak
outcast
outcome
outcry
outdid
outdo
outdoing
outdone
outdoor
outer
outermost
outfit
outfitter
outing
outlay
outlet

outline
outlook
outlying
outnumber
out-patient
output
outrageous
outright
outset
outside
outsize
outskirts
outspoken
outstanding
outward
ova
oval
ovalocyte
ovalocytosis
ovarian
ovariectomy
ovaries
ovary
ovation
oven
overall
overawe
overawed
overawing
overbearing
overcame
overcapacity
overcoat
overcome
overcoming
overcompensation
overcorrection
overdid
overdo
overdoing
overdone
overdose

overdraft
overdrawn
overdue
overexposure
overflow
overgrown
overheads
overhear
overheard
overhearing
overjoyed
overlap
overlapped
overlapping
overload
overlook
overpenetration
overpowering
overproduction
overran
overrate
overrated
overrating
overreach
overrun
overrunning
overseas
overshadow
oversight
overstep
overstepped
overstepping
oversubscribed
overt
overtake
overtaken
overtaking
overthrew
overthrow
overthrowing
overthrown
overtime

overtone
overtook
overwhelm
overwrought
Ovestin®
oviduct
Ovran®
Ovranette®
ovulation
ovulatory
ovum
Ovysmen®
owe
owed
owing
owner
oxaluria
oxamniquine
oxatomide
oxazepam
oxerutin
oxethazaine
oxidase
oxidation
oxide
oxidize
oxpentifylline
oxprenolol
oxybenzone
oxybuprocaine
oxycodone
oxygen
oxygenated
oxygenation
oxyhaemoglobin
oxymetazoline
oxymetholone
oxypertine
oxyphenbutazone
oxytetracycline
oxytocic
oxytocin

Oxyuris
oyster
ozone

Pp

32P
Pabrinex®
pace
paced
pacemaker
pacified
pacify
pacifying
pacing
package
packaging
packet
pact
pad
padded
padding
padimate O
padlock
paediatric
paediatrician
paediatrics
page
paged
Paget's disease
paging
paid
pail
pain
pained
painful
painfully
painless
painstaking
paint

painter
painting
pair
Palaprin Forte®
palatable
palatal
palate
palatine
palatoglossus
palatopharyngeus
pale
palette
palindromic
paling
palliate
palliation
palliative
pallid
pallor
palm
palmar
palmaris brevis
palmaris longus
palpable
palpably
palpate
palpation
palpebra
palpebrae
palpebral
palpitate
palpitation
palsy
paltry
Paludrine®
pamphlet
panacea
pancake
pancarditis
Pancoast's tumour
pancreas
Pancrease®

pancreatectomy
pancreatic
pancreatin
pancreatitis
pancreozymin
Pancrex®
pancuronium
pancytopenia
pandemic
pandemonium
pander
pane
panel
panelling
panencephalitis
pang
panhypopituitarism
panic
panicked
panicking
pannus
panoply
panorama
Panoxyl®
pansies
pansy
pant
panthenol
pantothenic
pantries
pantry
pants
papa
Papanicolaou's stain
  or smear
papaveretum
papaverine
paperback
paperweight
papier mâché
papilla
papillae

Pp

papillary
papillitis
papilloedema
papilloma
papillomata
papillomatosis
papillomatous
papular
papule
papulopustular
para-aortic
paracenteses
paracentesis
paracetamol
parachute
parachutist
paracolic
parade
paraded
parading
paradox
paradoxes
paradoxical
paradoxically
paraesthesia
paraffin
paragon
paragraph
parainfluenza virus
paraldehyde
parallax
parallel
paralyse
paralysed
paralysing
paralysis
paralytic
Paramax®
paramedian
paramedical
parameter
parametrium

paramount
paramyxovirus
paranasal
paranoia
paranoid
paraoesophageal
paraphernalia
paraphimosis
paraphrase
paraphrenia
paraphrenic
paraplegia
paraplegic
paraproteinaemia
paraproteins
parapsychology
paraquat
parasitaemia
parasitaemic
parasite
parasitic
parasiticidal
parasiticide
parasitology
parasuicide
parasympathetic
parasympathomimetic
parathormone
parathyroid
parathyroidectomy
paratracheal
paratyphoid
paravertebral
parboil
parcel
parcelled
parcelling
parch
parchment
pardon
pardonable
pare

pared
parenchyma
parenchymal
parenchymatous
parent
parentage
parental
parenteral
parenterally
parentheses
parenthesis
parenthetical
Parentrovite®
paresis
paretic
parietal
parieto-occipital
parietotemporal
paring
parish
parishes
parity
Parkinsonism
Parkinson's disease
parliament
parliamentary
Parlodel®
Parnate®
paronychia
parotidectomy
parotid gland
parotitis
parous
Paroven®
paroxysm
paroxysmal
pars
Parstelin®
partial
partiality
partially
participant

participate
participated
participating
participation
participle
particle
particular
particularly
particulate
parties
partisan
partition
partly
partner
partnership
parturition
party
pascal
Pascal
pass
passable
passage
passenger
passer-by
passers-by
passive
passivity
passport
password
pasta
paste
pastel
Pasteurella
pasteurization
pasteurize
pasteurized
pasteurizing
pasties
pastille
pastime
past pointing
pastries

pastry
pasty
pat
patch
patches
patchy
pate
pâté
patella
patellae
patellar
patellectomy
patency
patent
patently
paternal
paternally
paternity
Paterson-Kelly
   syndrome
path
pathetic
pathetically
pathogen
pathogenesis
pathogenetic
pathogenic
pathogenicity
pathognomonic
pathological
pathologically
pathologist
pathology
pathophysiological
pathophysiologically
pathophysiology
patience
patient
patrol
patrolled
patrolling
patron

patronize
patronized
patronizing
patted
pattern
patterned
patting
patulous
Paul-Bunnel reaction
   or test
paunch
paunches
pause
paused
pausing
Pavacol-D®
pavement
pavilion
Pavlov's pouch
pawnbroker
pay
payable
payee
paying
payment
payroll
pay-slip
peace
peaceable
peaceably
peaceful
peacefully
peach
peaches
peak
peak expiratory flow
   rate
peaky
peal
peau d'orange
pebble
peckish

Pp

pectineus
pectoral
pectoralis
pectoriloquy
pectus
pectus carinatum
pectus excavatum
peculiar
peculiarities
peculiarity
pedal
pedalled
pedalling
peddle
peddled
peddling
pedestal
pedestrian
pedicle
pediculosis
Pediculus
Pediculus capitis
Pediculus corporis
Pediculus pubis
pedigree
pedlar
pedometer
peduncle
peduncular
pedunculated
peel
peg
pegged
pegging
pejorative
Pel-Ebstein fever
pellagra
pellet
pell-mell
pelmet
pelvic
pelvimetry

pelvis
pemoline
pemphigoid
pemphigus
pemphigus vulgaris
pen
penalize
penalized
penalizing
penalties
penalty
penance
penbutolol
pence
pencil
pencilled
pencilling
pendant
pendent
pending
pendulous
penetrance
penetrate
penetrated
penetrating
penetration
penicillamine
penicillin
penicillinase
penicillin V
penicillin VK
penile
penis
Penject®
pen-name
penned
pennies
penniless
penning
penny
pension
pensioner

pensive
pentaerythritol
  tetranitrate
pentagastrin
pentagon
pentamidine
pentathlon
pentazocine
penthouse
pentose
pent-up
penultimate
people
peopled
peopling
Pepcid PM®
pepper
peppermint
pepsin
pepsinogen
peptic
peptidase
peptides
perborate
perceive
perceived
perceiving
per cent
percentage
perceptible
perceptibly
perception
perceptive
percolate
percolated
percolating
percolation
percolator
percussion
percutaneous
perennial
perennially

perfect
perfection
perfectionist
perforate
perforated
perforating
perforation
perform
performance
perfuse
perfusion
Pergonal®
perhaps
Periactin®
perianal
periarterial
periarteritis
periarticular
pericardectomy
pericardial
pericardiocentesis
pericarditis
pericardium
pericranium
pericyazine
peril
perilous
perilymph
perimeter
perinatal
perineal
perineorrhaphy
perinephric
perineum
period
periodic
periodical
periodically
periodicity
periodontal
perioperative
perioral

periosteal
periosteum
periostitis
peripatetic
peripheral
peripheries
periphery
periportal
perish
perishable
peristalsis
peristaltic
peritoneal
peritoneum
peritonitis
peritonsillar
periumbilical
perk
perlingual
permanence
permanency
permanent
permanganate
permeability
permeable
permeate
permeated
permeating
permeation
permissible
permission
permissive
permit
permitted
permitting
permutation
pernasal
pernicious
peroneal
peroneus
peroneus brevis
peroneus longus

peroneus tertius
peroxide
perpendicular
perpetrate
perpetrated
perpetrating
perpetrator
perpetual
perpetually
perpetuate
perpetuated
perpetuating
perphenazine
perplex
perplexities
perplexity
perquisite
Persantin®
per se
persecute
persecuted
persecuting
persecution
persecutor
perseverance
perseveration
persevere
persevered
persevering
persist
persistence
persistent
person
persona
personable
personal
personalities
personality
personally
personification
personified
personify

Pp

personifying
personnel
perspective
Perspex®
perspiration
perspire
perspired
perspiring
persuade
persuaded
persuading
persuasion
persuasive
persulphate
pertaining
Perthes' disease
pertinent
Pertofran®
perturb
pertussis
perusal
pervade
pervaded
pervading
pervenous
perverse
perversion
perversity
pervert
pes
pes cavus
pes planus
pessary
pessimism
pessimist
pessimistic
pessimistically
pesticide
pestilence
pestis
pestle
petal

petechia
petechiae
petechial
pethidine
petite
petition
petit mal
Petri dish
petroleum
petrosal
petrous
petticoat
petulant
Peutz-Jeghers
 syndrome
pewter
Peyer's patches
Peyronie's disease
Pfannenstiel's incision
pH
phaeochromocytoma
phage
phage-typing
phagocyte
phagocytic
phagocytosis
phalangeal
phalanges
phalanx
phallic
phallus
phantom
pharmaceutical
pharmacies
pharmacist
pharmacokinetics
pharmacological
pharmacologically
pharmacologist
pharmacology
pharmacopoeia
pharmacopoeial

pharmacy
pharyngal
pharyngectomy
pharyngitis
pharynx
Phasal®
phase
phased
phasing
phenazocine
phenazone
phenelzine
Phenergan®
phenethicillin
phenindamine
phenindione
pheniramine
phenobarbitone
phenol
phenolic
phenolphthalein
phenomena
phenomenal
phenomenon
phenoperidine
phenothiazine
phenotype
phenotypical
phenoxybenzamine
phenoxymethyl·
 penicillin
phentermine
phentolamine
phenyl
phenylbutazone
phenylephrine
phenylketonuria
 (PKU)
phenylpropanolamine
phenytoin
phial
philanthropy

philately
philosophy
phimosis
pHiso-MED®
phlebitis
phlebolith
phlebotomist
phlebotomy
phlegm
phlegmatic
phlyctenular
phlyctenule
phobia
phobias
phobic
phocomelia
pholcodine
phonation
phone
phonetics
phoney
phonocardiogram
phonocardiograph
phonocardiography
phony
phosgene
phosphatase
phosphate
phosphaturia
phospholipid
phosphonates
phosphonecrosis
phosphorescent
phosphorous
phosphorus
phosphorylases
phosphorylation
photochemical
photocoagulation
photocopied
photocopy
photocopying

photodermatoses
photodermatosis
photograph
photographer
photographic
photographically
photography
photometer
photometry
photomicrograph
photophobia
photophobic
photosensitive
photosensitization
phototherapy
phrase
phrased
phrasing
phrenetic
phrenic
phrenology
phthisis
Phyllocontin
  Continus®
Physeptone®
physical
physically
physician
physicist
physics
physiological
physiologically
physiologist
physiology
physiotherapist
physiotherapy
physique
physostigmine
phytase
phytate
Phytex®
phytic acid

phytomenadione
pia mater
pica
picket
picketing
Pick's disease
Pickwickian syndrome
picnic
picnicking
pico-
picogram
Picolax®
picornavirus
picosulphate
picture
piebald
piece
piecemeal
piecework
pierce
pierced
piercing
Pierre Robin
  syndrome
pigeon chest
pigeon-hole
piggy-back
pigment
pigmentation
pigtail
pile
piled
piles
pileum
pilgrimage
pili
piling
pillar
pillion
pillow
pilocarpine
pilonidal

Pp

pilosebaceous
pilot
Pimafucin®
pimozide
pimple
pimply
pin
pinafore
pincers
pinch
pinched
pinches
pindolol
pineal
pineapple
pinguecula
pink
pinna
pinnacle
pinned
pinning
pint
pinta
pinworm
pioneer
pioneered
pioneering
pipe
piped
pipeline
pipenzolate
piperacillin
piperazine
piperazine oestrone
  sulphate
pipette
piping
pipothiazine palmitate
Piptalin®
piquant
pique
piqued

piquing
pirate
pirbuterol
pirenzepine
piretanide
piriform
piriformis
Piriton®
piroxicam
pisiform
pistol
piston
pit
pitch
pitcher
pitches
piteous
pitfall
pitiable
pitied
pitiful
pitifully
Pitressin®
pitted
pitting
pituitary
pity
pitying
pityriasis
pityriasis capitis
pityriasis rosea
pityriasis versicolor
Pityrosporum
pivampicillin
pivmecillinam
pivot
pizotifen
placard
placate
placated
placating
place

placebo
placed
placenta
placental
placenta praevia
placentography
placid
placing
plague
plain
plan
plane
planet
planetary
plankton
planned
planning
plantar
plantar fascittis
plantar flexion
plantaris
planter
plaque
Plaquenil®
plasma
plasmacyte
plasmacytoma
plasmapheresis
plasmin
plasminogen
plasmodial
Plasmodium
plasmolysis
plaster
plaster of Paris
plastic
Plasticine®
plasticity
plate
plateau
plateaus
plateaux

plated
platelet
platform
plating
platinum
platyhelminth
platysma
platysmal
plausibility
plausible
plausibly
playful
playfully
playschool
plead
pleasant
pleasantness
pleasantries
pleasantry
please
pleased
pleasing
pleasurable
pleasurably
pleasure
pledge
pledged
pledget
pledging
plenary
plenteous
plentiful
plentifully
plenty
pleomorphic
pleomorphism
plethora
plethoric
plethysmograph
plethysmographic
plethysmography
pleura

pleural
pleurectomy
pleurisy
pleuritic
pleurocentesis
pleurodesis
pleurodynia
plexus
pliable
pliant
plica
plicamycin
plicate
plication
plied
pliers
plight
plug
plugged
plugging
plumbism
plume
Plummer-Vinson
  syndrome
plummet
plunge
plunged
plunging
pluriglandular
plus
plutonium
ply
plying
pneumatic
pneumatically
pneumatization
pneumaturia
pneumococcal
pneumococcus
pneumoconioses
pneumoconiosis
Pneumocystis carinii

pneumoencephalo·
  gram
pneumoencephalo·
  graphy
pneumomediastinum
pneumonectomy
pneumonia
pneumonic
pneumonitis
pneumoperitoneum
pneumothorax
poach
pockmark
podalic version
podophyllin
podophyllum resin
poganiasis
poikilocyte
poikilocytosis
point
pointed
pointer
pointing
pointless
poised
poison
poisoning
poisonous
poke
poked
poking
polar
polarimeter
polarimetry
polarity
polarization
polarize
polarized
poldine
  methylsulphate
police
policed

policeman
policemen
policies
policing
policy
polio
polioencephalitis
poliomyelitis
polio virus
polish
polishes
polite
politely
politeness
politic
political
politically
politician
politics
Politzer's bag
pollen
pollute
polluted
polluting
pollution
polyamide
Polya operation
polyarteritis
polyarteritis nodosa
polyarthralgia
polyarthritis
polyarthropathy
Polycrol®
polycystic
polycythaemia
polydactyly
polydipsia
polyestradiol
polygeline
polygraph
polyhydramnios
polymorph

polymorphic
polymorphism
polymorphonuclear
polymorphous
polymyalgia
  rheumatica
polymyositis
polymyxin
polymyxin B
polyneuritis
polyneuropathy
polynoxylin
polyoma
polyp
polypectomy
polypeptide
polypharmacy
polypi
polypoid
polyposis
polyposis coli
polypus
polysaccharidase
polysaccharide
polystyrene
Polytar®
polytechnic
polythene
polythiazide
Polytrim®
polyurethane
polyuria
polyvinyl alcohol
pomegranate
pompholyx
Ponderax®
ponies
pons
Ponstan®
pontine
pony
pony-trekking

popliteal
popliteus
poppies
poppy
populace
popular
popularity
popularize
popularized
popularizing
populate
populated
populating
population
populous
pore
pored
poring
porosity
porous
porphobilinogen
porphyria
porphyria cutanea
  tarda
porphyria variegata
porphyrin
porphyrinuria
portable
portacaval
porta hepatis
portal circulation
portal hypertension
portal vein
portent
porter
portion
portly
portmanteau
portmanteaus
portmanteaux
portocaval
portrait

portray
portrayal
Portuguese
Posalfilin®
pose
posed
posing
position
positive
positively
positive pressure
  ventilation
possess
possession
possessive
possessor
posseting
possibilities
possibility
possible
possum
postage
postal
postanaesthetic
postauricular
postcard
postcentral
postcoital
postconcussional
postencephalitic
postepileptic
poster
poste restante
posterior
posterity
postganglionic
postgastrectomy
postherpetic
posthumous
postictal
postmature
postmaturity

postmenopausal
postmortem
postmyocardial
  infarction syndrome
postnasal
postnatal
postnatally
postoperative
postoperatively
postpartum
postpone
postponed
postponement
postponing
postprandial
postscript
postulate
postural
posture
postwar
potable
potash
potassium
potassium-sparing
potato
potatoes
potency
potent
potential
potentially
potion
Pott's disease or
  fracture
pouch
pouches
pouch of Douglas
poultice
poultry
pound
pour
poverty
povidone-iodine

powder
powdery
power
powered
powerful
powerfully
powerless
pox
pox virus
practicable
practical
practically
practice
practise
practised
practising
practitioner
practolol
Prader-Willi syndrome
praecox
praevia
pragmatism
praise
praised
praising
pralidoxime mesylate
pramoxine
prandial
prawn
Praxilene®
pray
prayer
prazepam
praziquantel
prazosin
preach
preamble
preanaesthetic
prearrange
prearranged
prearranging
precancerous

precarious
precaution
precautionary
precede
preceded
precedence
precedent
preceding
precept
precinct
precious
precipitate
precipitated
precipitating
precipitation
precipitin
precise
precisely
precision
preclude
precluded
precluding
precognition
preconception
preconceptual
precordial
precordium
precursor
predecessor
Predenema®
Predfoam®
predicament
predict
predictable
predictably
prediction
predilection
predispose
predisposition
prednisolone
prednisone
predominant

Predsol®
pre-eclampsia
pre-eclamptic
pre-eminent
prefabricated
preface
prefer
preferable
preference
preferential
preferred
preferring
Prefil®
prefix
prefixes
prefrontal
Pregaday®
preganglionic
pregnancies
pregnancy
pregnanediol
pregnanetriol
pregnant
prehensile
prejudge
prejudged
prejudging
prejudice
prejudiced
prejudicial
prejudicing
preliminaries
preliminary
prelude
premalignant
Premarin®
premature
prematurely
premedication
premeditated
premenstrual
premise

premises
premium
premiums
premolars
premonition
premorbid
Prempak®
prenylamine
preoccupation
preoccupied
preoperative
preoperatively
prepaid
preparalytic
preparation
preparatory
prepare
prepared
preparing
prepatellar
prepay
prepaying
prepayment
preponderance
prepossessing
preposterous
prepubertal
prepuce
preputial
prepyloric
prerenal
prerequisite
prerogative
presbycousis
presbyopia
presbyopic
prescribe
prescribed
prescribing
prescription
presence
presenile dementia

present
presentable
presentably
presentation
presentiment
presently
preservation
preservative
preserve
preserved
preserving
preside
presided
presidency
president
presiding
pressor
pressure
pressurize
pressurized
pressurizing
Prestel®
prestige
prestigious
presumably
presume
presumed
presuming
presumption
presumptuous
pretence
pretend
pretentious
pretext
pretibial
prevail
prevalence
prevalent
prevent
preventive
preview
previous

Priadel®
priapism
price
priced
priceless
pricing
prick
prickle
prickled
prickling
prickly
prickly heat
pride
prided
priding
pried
prilocaine
Primalan®
primaquine
primarily
primary
Primaxin®
primidone
primigravida
primigravidae
primipara
primiparous
primitive
Primolut®
primordial
princeps
principal
principalities
principality
principally
principle
P-R interval
Prioderm®
priorities
priority
Pripsen®
prism

prisoner
pristine
privacy
private
privately
privatization
privilege
privileged
prize
prized
prizing
Pro-Actidil®
probabilities
probability
probable
probably
proband
Pro-Banthine®
probation
probe
probed
probenecid
probing
problem
problematic
probucol
procainamide
procaine
procarbazine
procedure
proceed
proceeds
process
processes
procession
processus
prochlorperazine
procidentia
proclaim
proclamation
procreate
procreation

Pp

proctalgia
proctitis
proctocolectomy
proctocolitis
Proctofoam®
proctoscope
proctoscopic
proctoscopy
Proctosedyl®
procuration
procurator fiscal
procure
procured
procuring
procyclidine
prodigious
prodromal
prodrome
pro-drug
produce
produced
producer
producing
product
production
productive
productively
productivity
Profasi®
profess
profession
professional
professionally
professor
proffer
proficiency
proficient
profile
profit
profitable
profitably
profited

profiting
profit-sharing
proflavine
profound
profunda
profunda brachii
profunda femoris
profuse
profusely
profusion
progeria
Progestasert®
progestational
progesterone
progestogen
progestogen-only
prognosis
prognostic
prognosticate
program
programmable
programme
programmed
programming
progress
progression
progressive
progressively
proguanil
Progynova®
prohibit
prohibited
prohibiting
prohibition
prohibitive
project
projectile
projection
projector
prolactin
prolactinoma
prolapse

proliferate
proliferated
proliferating
proliferation
proliferative
prolific
proline
prolintane
prolong
promazine
promethazine
prominence
prominent
promise
promised
promises
promising
promontory
promote
promoted
promoter
promoting
promotion
prompt
promptly
pronate
pronation
pronator
pronator quadratus
pronator teres
prone
pronounce
pronounced
pronouncement
pronouncing
pronunciation
Propaderm®
propaganda
propagandist
propagate
propagated
propagating

propagation
propagator
propamidine
  isethionate
propantheline
proper
properties
property
prophylactic
prophylactically
prophylaxis
Propine®
propionic acid
propofol
proportion
proportional
proportionally
proportionate
proportionately
proposal
propose
proposed
proposing
proposition
propranolol
proprietary
proprietory
proprioceptive
proprioceptor
proptosis
propyl
propylthiouracil
pro rata
prose
prosecute
prosecuted
prosecuting
prosecution
Prosobee®
prospect
prospective
prospectus

prospectuses
prostaglandin
prostate
prostatectomy
prostatic
prostatism
prostatitis
prostheses
prosthesis
prosthetic
prosthetics
Prostigmin®
Prostin®
prostrate
prostrated
prostrating
prostration
protagonist
protamine
Protaphane®
protease
protect
protection
protective
protector
protégé
protein
proteinase
protein-binding
proteinuria
proteolysis
proteolytic
protest
Protestant
Proteus
Prothiaden®
prothionamide
prothrombin
protirelin
protocol
proton
protoplasm

protoplasmic
protoporphyria
protoporphyrin
prototype
protozoa
protozoal
protozoon
protract
protractor
protriptyline
protrude
protruded
protruding
protrusio acetabuli
protrusion
protuberance
protuberant
proud
prove
proved
Pro-Vent®
Provera®
proverbial
proverbially
provide
provided
providing
province
provincial
provincially
proving
provision
provisional
provisionally
proviso
provisos
provocation
provoke
provoked
provoking
prowess
prowl

prowler
proxies
proximal
proximally
proximity
proxy
proxymetacaine
prudent
prune belly syndrome
prurigo
pruritic
pruritus
pruritus ani
pruritus vulvae
prussic acid
prying
pseudobulbar
pseudocholinesterase
pseudocyesis
pseudocyst
pseudodementia
pseudoephedrine
pseudofracture
pseudogout
pseudohermaphrodite
pseudohermaphroditis
pseudohermaphro·
 ditism
pseudohypoparathyro·
 idism
pseudomembranous
pseudomembranous
 colitis
Pseudomonas
Pseudomonas
 aeruginosa
Pseudomonas
 pyocanea
pseudomonic
pseudoparalysis
pseudopodia
pseudopodium

pseudopolyposis
pseudoxanthoma
pseudoxanthoma
 elasticum
psittacosis
psoas
psoralen
psoriasis
psoriatic
psyche
psychiatric
psychiatrist
psychiatry
psychic
psychical
psychoanalyse
psychoanalysis
psychoanalyst
psychoanalytic
psychodrama
psychodynamics
psychogenic
psychogeriatric
psychological
psychologically
psychologist
psychology
psychometry
psychomotor
psychoneurosis
psychoneurotic
psychopath
psychopathic
psychopathological
psychopathologically
psychopathology
psychopathy
psychopharmacology
psychoses
psychosexual
psychosis
psychosomatic

psychosurgery
psychotherapeutic
psychotherapy
psychotic
psychotropic
pterygial
pterygium
pterygoid
ptosis
ptyalin
ptyalism
pubertal
puberty
pubescent
pubic
pubis
public
publication
publicity
publicly
pudendal block
pudendum
Pudenz-Hayer valve
puerile
puerperal
puerperium
puffiness
puffy
pulley
pulleys
Pulmadil®
Pulmicort®
pulmonary
pulsate
pulsated
pulsatile
pulsating
pulsation
pulse
pulsed
pulseless
pulsing

pulsus
pulsus alternans
pulsus bigeminus
pulsus paradoxus
pulverization
pumice stone
punch drunk
puncta
punctate
punctual
punctuality
punctually
punctuate
punctuated
punctuating
punctuation
punctum
puncture
punctured
puncturing
punish
punishable
punishment
pupa
pupae
pupil
pupillary
purchase
purchased
purchaser
purchasing
pure
purée
purely
purgation
purgative
purgatory
purge
purged
purging
purification
purified

purified protein
  derivative (PPD)
purify
purifying
purine
Purkinje's fibres
purpose
purposeful
purposefully
purposely
purpura
pursue
pursued
pursuer
pursuing
pursuit
purulent
pus
pustular
pustule
put
putamen
putrefaction
putrefy
putrefying
putrid
putrified
putting
putty
PUVA
puzzle
puzzled
puzzling
pyaemia
pyaemic
pyelitis
pyelogram
pyelography
pyeloilithotomy
pyelonephritis
pyjamas
pyknic

pyknosis
pyknotic
pylon
pyloric
pyloroplasty
pylorospasm
pylorus
pyoderma
pyogenic
pyometra
pyonephrosis
pyopneumothorax
pyorrhoea
pyorrhoea alveolaris
pyorrhoeal
pyosalpinx
pyothorax
pyramid
pyramidal
pyramidalis
pyrantel
pyrazinamide
Pyrex®
pyrexia
pyrexial
pyridostigmine
pyridoxine
pyrimethamine
pyrimidine
pyrithione
Pyrogastrone®
pyrogen
pyrogenic
pyromania
pyuria

Qq

Q-fever
Q-T interval
quad
quadrangle
quadrant
quadrantanopia
quadratus
quadratus femoris
quadratus lumborum
quadriceps
quadrilateral
quadriplegia
quadriplegic
quadruped
quadruple
quadruplet
quaff
qualification
qualified
qualify
qualifying
qualitative
qualities
quality
qualm
quandaries
quandary
quango
quangos
quantitative
quantities
quantity
quantum
quarantine
quarrel
quarrelled
quarrelling
quarrelsome

quarried
quarries
quarry
quarrying
quart
quartan
quarter
quarterly
quartz
quash
quasi-
quaternary
quaternary ammonium
quay
queasily
queasiness
queasy
Queckenstedt's test
queen
queer
quell
Quellada®
quench
queried
queries
query
querying
quest
question
questionnaire
Questran®
queue
queued
queueing
queuing
quick
quicken
quickening
quickness
Quicksol®
quid
quid pro quo

quiescent
quiet
quieten
quietness
quill
quilt
quin
quinalbarbitone
quinidine
quinine
Quinoderm®
quinolone
quinsy
quintessence
quintessential
quintet
quintuplet
quire
quirk
quit
quite
quitted
quitting
quiver
quiz
quizzed
quizzes
quizzical
quizzically
quizzing
quorum
quota
quotas
quotation
quote
quoted
quotient
quoting

Rr

rabbi
rabbis
rabbit
rabid
rabies
race
racecourse
rachitic
racial
racially
racism
racist
rack
racket
racquet
racy
rad
radar
radial
radialis
radiance
radiant
radiate
radiated
radiating
radiation
radiator
radical
radically
radicular
radiculogram
radiculography
radii
radio
radioactive
radioactivity
radioed
radiograph

radiographer
radiographic
radiography
radio-immunoassay
radioing
radio-iodine
radio-isotope
radiological
radiologically
radiologist
radiology
radiolucency
radiolucent
radionuclide
radiopacity
radiopaque
radioresistant
radios
radiosensitive
radiosensitivity
radiotherapist
radiotherapy
radio-ulnar
radium
radius
radon seed
rage
raged
raging
raid
raider
rail
railing
railway
rain
rainbow
rainy
raise
raised
raisin
raising
râle

rallied
rallies
rally
rallying
rami
ramification
ramify
ramp
Ramsay Hunt
  syndrome
Ramstedt's operation
ramus
ran
ranch
ranches
rancid
random
rang
range
ranged
ranging
ranitidine
rank
ransack
rant
ranula
ranular
rapacious
rape
raped
raphe
rapid
rapidity
raping
Rapitard MC®
rapturous
rare
rarefaction
rarefied
rarely
raring
rarities

rarity
rash
rashes
rasp
raspberries
raspberry
RAST
rat-bite fever
ratchet
rate
rateable
rated
rather
Rathke's pouch
ratification
ratified
ratify
ratifying
rating
ratio
ration
rational
rationale
rationalization
rationalize
rationalized
rationalizing
rationally
rationed
rationing
ratios
rattle
rattled
rattlesnake
rattling
raucous
rauwolfia
ravenous
ravine
ravishing
Raynaud's disease or
  syndrome

razor
razoxane
re
reach
react
reaction
reactionary
reactivate
reactivation
reactivity
reactor
read
reader
readily
readiness
reading
ready
reagent
reagin
realist
realistic
realistically
realities
reality
reality orientation
  (RO)
realization
realize
realized
realizing
really
realm
rearguard
rearrangement
reason
reasonable
reasonably
reasoned
reasoning
reassurance
reassure
reassured

reassuring
rebate
rebel
rebelled
rebelling
rebellion
rebellious
rebound
rebreathing
rebuff
rebuke
rebuked
rebuking
rebut
rebuttal
rebutted
rebutting
recalcitrance
recalcitrant
recall
recannulation
recap
recapitulate
recapitulated
recapitulating
recapitulation
recapped
recapping
recapture
recaptured
recapturing
recede
receded
receding
receipt
receive
received
receiver
receiving
recent
recently
receptacle

reception
receptionist
receptive
receptor
recess
recesses
recession
recessive
recipe
recipient
reciprocal
reciprocally
reciprocate
reciprocated
reciprocating
reckless
Recklinghausen's
  disease
reckon
reclaim
reclamation
recline
reclined
reclining
recognition
recognizable
recognizably
recognize
recognized
recognizing
recoil
recollect
recollection
recombinant DNA
recombination
recommend
recommendation
recompense
reconcile
reconciled
reconciliation
reconciling

reconnaissance
reconstituted
record
recorder
recount
recoup
recourse
recover
recovered
recovering
recovery
re-creation
recreation
recrimination
recrudescence
recruit
recruitment
rectal
rectally
rectangle
rectangular
rectified
rectify
rectifying
rectocele
rectosigmoid
rectosigmoidectomy
rectouterine
rectovaginal
rectum
rectus abdominis
rectus femoris
recumbency
recumbent
recuperate
recuperated
recuperating
recuperation
recuperative
recur
recurred
recurrence

recurrent
recurring
redden
redeem
redeemable
redeeming
redemption
redeploy
Redeptin®
red-handed
redolent
redouble
redoubled
redoubling
redoubtable
redress
reduce
reduced
reducible
reducing
reductase
reduction
redundancies
redundancy
redundant
reduplicated
reduplication
re-education
re-entry
refectories
refectory
refer
referee
reference
referenda
referendum
referendums
referred
referred pain
referring
refine
refined

refinement
refineries
refinery
refining
reflation
reflect
reflection
reflective
reflector
reflex
reflexive
reflux
reform
reformation
reformer
refract
refraction
refractive
refractory
refrain
refresh
refresher course
refreshment
refrigeration
refrigerator
refund
refusal
refuse
refused
refusing
refute
refuted
refuting
regain
Regaine®
regard
regarding
regardless
regenerate
regeneration
régime
regimen

regiment
regimentation
region
regional
regional ileitis
regionally
register
registrar
registries
registry
regression
regressive
regret
regretful
regretfully
regrettable
regrettably
regretted
regretting
Regulan®
regular
regularity
regulate
regulated
regulating
regulation
regulator
regurgitate
regurgitated
regurgitating
regurgitation
rehabilitate
rehabilitated
rehabilitating
rehabilitation
rehearsal
Rehibin®
Rehidrat®
rehydration
reign
reimburse
reimbursed

reimbursing
reimplantation
rein
reinfection
reinforce
reinforced
reinforcement
reinforcements
reinforcing
reinstate
reinstated
reinstatement
reinstating
reinsurance
reiterate
reiterated
reiterating
reiteration
reiterative
Reiter's syndrome
reject
rejection
rejoinder
rejuvenate
rejuvenated
rejuvenating
relapse
relapsed
relapsing
relapsing fever
relate
related
relating
relation
relationship
relative
relatively
relax
relaxant
relaxation
relay
release

released
releasing
relegate
relegated
relegating
relegation
relent
relentless
relevance
relevant
reliable
reliably
reliance
reliant
relied
relief
relieve
relieved
relieving
relinquish
reluctance
reluctant
rely
relying
remain
remainder
remark
remarkable
remarkably
remedial
remedied
remedies
remedy
remedying
remember
remembered
remembering
remembrance
remind
reminder
reminisce
reminisced

reminiscence
reminiscent
reminiscing
remiss
remission
remit
remittance
remitted
remittent
remitting
remorse
remote
remotely
removal
remove
removed
removing
REM sleep
remunerate
remunerated
remunerating
remuneration
remunerative
renal
Rendells®
render
rendezvous
renew
renewal
renin
rennin
renounce
renounced
renouncing
renovate
renovated
renovating
renovation
renowned
renunciation
reorganization
reorganize

reorganized
reorganizing
reo virus
repaid
repair
repaired
repairing
reparation
repay
repaying
repayment
repeal
repeat
repeatability
repeatedly
repel
repellant
repelled
repellent
repelling
repent
repentant
repercussion
repertoire
repetition
repetitious
repetitive
replace
replaced
replacement
replacing
replenish
replete
replica
replicas
replied
replies
reply
replying
repolarization
report
reporter

repose
repositories
repository
reprehensible
reprehensibly
represent
representation
representative
repress
repression
repressive
repressor
reprieve
reprieved
reprieving
reprimand
reprisal
reproach
reproaches
reproachful
reproachfully
reproduce
reproduced
reproducing
reproduction
reproductive
reproterol
reptile
reptilian
republic
repudiate
repudiated
repudiating
repudiation
repugnant
repulsion
repulsive
reputable
reputation
repute
request
require

required
requirement
requiring
requisite
requisition
rescind
rescue
rescued
rescuing
research
researcher
researches
resect
resectable
resection
resectoscope
resemblance
resemble
resembled
resembling
resent
reserpine
reservation
reserve
reserved
reserving
reservoir
reshaping
reside
resided
residence
resident
residential
residing
residual
residue
residuum
resign
resignation
resilient
resin
resinous

resin-uptake
resist
resistance
resolute
resolution
resolve
resolved
resolving
resonance
resonant
resonator
Resonium®
Resonium A®
resorcinol
resorption
resort
resounding
resource
resourceful
respect
respectability
respectable
respectably
respectful
respectfully
respective
respiration
respirator
respiratory
respiratory distress
    syndrome (RDS)
respiratory syncytial
    virus (RSV)
respirometer
resplendent
respond
response
responsibilities
responsibility
responsible
responsibly
responsive

restaurant
restitution
restive
restless
restoration
restorative
restore
restored
restoring
restrain
restraint
restrict
restriction
restrictive
result
resultant
resume
résumé
resumed
resuming
resumption
resurgent
resurrect
resurrection
resuscitate
resuscitated
resuscitating
resuscitation
resuscitative
resuture
retail
retailer
retain
retainer
retaliate
retaliated
retaliating
retaliation
retardation
retarded
retch
retching

rete
retention
retentive
rete testis
reticence
reticent
reticular
reticulin
reticulocyte
reticulocytoma
reticulocytosis
reticuloendothelial
  system (RES)
reticulum
retina
Retin-A®
retinaculum
retinae
retinal
retinitis
retinitis pigmentosa
retinoblastoma
retinol
retinopathy
retinoscope
retinoscopy
retinue
retiral
retire
retired
retirement
retiring
retort
retrace
retraced
retracing
retract
retractable
retractile
retraction
retractor
retreat

retribution
retrieve
retrieved
retrieving
retrobulbar
retrobulbar neuritis
retrocaecal
retrocardiac
retroflexion
retrograde
retrolental fibroplasia
retro-ocular
retroperitoneal
retropharyngeal
retroplacental
retropubic
retrospect
retrospection
retrospective
retrosternal
retrotracheal
retroversion
retroverted
Retrovir®
return
returnable
reunion
reunite
reunited
reuniting
reusable
revaluation
revascularization
revascularize
reveal
revelation
revenge
revenged
revenging
revenue
reverberate
reverberated

reverberating
reverberation
reversal
reverse
reversed
reversible
reversing
reversion
revert
revise
revised
revising
revision
revitalization
revival
revive
revived
reviving
revoke
revoked
revoking
revolt
revolting
revolution
revolutionaries
revolutionary
revolutionize
revolutionized
revolutionizing
revolve
revolved
revolving
revulsion
reward
Reye's syndrome
rhabdomyoma
rhabdomyosarcoma
rhabdosarcoma
Rhabdovirus
rheoscope
rheostat
Rhesus

Rhesus factor
Rhesus
  isoimmunization
rhetoric
rhetorical
rhetorically
rheumatic
rheumatism
rheumatoid
rheumatology
Rheumox®
rhinencephalon
rhinitis
rhinitis
  medicamentosa
Rhinocort®
rhinophyma
rhinoplasty
rhinorrhoea
rhinoscopic
rhinoscopy
Rhinosporidium
rhinovirus
rhizotomy
rhodopsin
rhomboid
rhonchus
rhubarb
rhyme
rhymed
rhyming
rhythm
rhythmic
rhythmical
rhythmically
ribavirin
ribbed
ribbon
riboflavine
ribonuclease
ribonucleic acid (RNA)
ribosome

rice
rice-water stool
rich
riches
richness
rickets
Rickettsia
rickettsial
rickety
rickety rosary
ricochet
rid
riddance
ridden
ridding
riddle
riddled
riddling
ride
rider
ridge
ridiculous
riding
Riedel's thyroiditis
rifampicin
rig
rigged
rigging
right
rightful
rightfully
rigid
rigidity
rigor
rigor mortis
rigorous
rigour
Rimactazid®
rimiterol
rind
ring
ringed

Ringer's solution
ringing
ringworm
rink
Rinne's test
rinse
rinsed
rinsing
rioter
rip
ripe
ripen
ripped
ripping
rise
risen
rising
risk
rissole
risus sardonicus
ritodrine
ritual
ritually
rivalry
rivet
riveted
riveting
Rivotril®
rivulet
Roaccutane®
road
roast
rob
Robaxin 750®
robbed
robberies
robbery
robbing
robe
robust
rocky
rode

rodent
rodent ulcer
roentgen
rogue
roguish
rôle
roll
Roman
Romanian
Romanovsky's stain
romantic
romantically
Romberg's sign
Ronicol®
roof
roofs
roomy
root
rope
roped
roping
Rorschach test
rosacea
rose
rose bengal
roseola
Roseola infantum
rosette
rosoxacin
roster
rostra
rostrum
rostrums
rosy
rot
rota
Rotacaps®
Rotahaler®
rotary
rotas
rotate
rotated

rotating
rotation
rotator
rotavirus
Rotersept®
Roth spots
rotted
rotten
rotting
rotund
rough
roughage
roughen
rouleaux
round
roundworm
rouse
roused
rousing
Rous' sarcoma virus
route
routine
routinely
Roux-en-Y operation
row
rowed
rowing
royal
royally
royalties
royalty
rub
rubbed
rubber
rubbing
rubbish
rubble
rubefacient
rubella
rubies
rubor
ruby

rude
rudimentary
rudiments
ruga
rugae
rugose
ruin
ruinous
rule
ruled
ruler
ruling
Rumanian
rumination
rumour
rump
rumpus
run
rung
runner
runners-up
runner-up
running
runway
rupture
ruptured
rupturing
rural
ruse
russet
Russian
rust
ruthless
ruthlessness
rutoside
rye
Ryle's tube
Rynacrom®

Ss

sabotage
Sabouraud's culture
  medium
sac
saccharide
saccharin
saccharine
saccular
sacculated
sacculation
saccule
sachet
sack
sacral
sacralization
sacred
sacrifice
sacrificed
sacrificing
sacroanterior
sacrococcygeal
sacroiliac
sacroiliitis
sacrolumbar
sacroposterior
sacrum
sad
sadder
saddest
saddle nose
sadism
sadist
sadistic
sadness
sadomasochism
sadomasochistic
safe
safeguard

safety
saga
sagacity
sage
sagittal
said
sail
sake
Salactol®
salaries
salary
Salazopyrin®
salbutamol
salcatonin
sale
salesman
salicylate
salicylic acid
salient
saline
saliva
salivary
salivate
salivated
salivating
salivation
Salk vaccine
sallow
Salmonella
Salmonella typhi
Salmonella
  typhimurium
salmonellosis
salpingectomy
salpingitis
salpingogram
salpingographic
salpingography
salpingo-
  oophorectomy
salpingostomy
salpinx

salsalate
salt
salvage
salvaged
salvaging
salvation
salve
salved
salving
sal volatile
Samaritans
same
sample
sampled
sampler
sampling
sanatoria
sanatorium
sanatoriums
sanction
sanctuaries
sanctuary
sand
sandfly
Sandimmun®
Sandocal®
Sando-K®
sandwich
sandwiches
sandy
sane
sang
sanguine
sanguineous
sanitary
sanitation
sanity
sank
Sanomigran®
sap
saphenous
saponification

sapped
sapping
saprophyte
saprophytic
sarcastic
sarcastically
sarcoid
sarcoidosis
sarcolemma
sarcoma
sarcomata
sarcomatosis
sarcomatous
Sarcoptes
sartorius
sat
satellite
satellitism
satiate
satiated
satiating
satirical
satirically
satisfaction
satisfactorily
satisfactory
satisfied
satisfy
satisfying
saturate
saturated
saturating
saturation
Saturday
sauce
sausage
savage
savagery
save
saved
saving
savings

saw
sawed
sawing
sawn
say
saying
scab
scabby
scabies
scabious
scaffolding
scald
scale
scalene
scalenus
scalp
scalpel
scaly
scan
scandal
scandalous
scanned
scanner
scanning
scant
scaphoid
scapula
scapular
scar
scarce
scarcely
scarcities
scarcity
scare
scared
scarf
scarfs
scarification
scaring
scarlatina
scarlatiniform
scarlet fever

scarred
scarring
scarves
scathing
scent
sceptic
sceptical
sceptically
scepticism
schedule
schema
schematic
scheme
schemed
scheming
Schering PC4®
Scheriproct®
Scheuermann's
 disease
Schick test
Schiff's reagent
Schilling test
Schirmer's test
schism
schistocyte
Schistosoma
schistosomiasis
schistosomicide
schizoid
schizophrenia
schizophreniac
schizophrenic
Schlatter's disease
Schlemm's canal
schleroderma
Schmorl's body or
 node
scholar
scholarship
school
Schwann's cell
Schwartze's operation

Schwartzmann
 reaction
sciatic
sciatica
science
scientific
scientifically
scientist
scintillography
scirrhous
scirrhus
scissor
scissors
sclera
scleral
scleritis
sclerocorneal
sclerodactylia
sclerodactyly
scleroderma
scleromalacia
 perforans
sclerosant
sclerose
sclerosis
sclerotherapy
sclerotic
sclerous
scoff
scold
scolex
scoliosis
scoliotic
scope
scopolamine
scorch
score
scored
scoring
scorn
scornful
scornfully

scorpion
scotoma
scotomata
scour
scourge
scourged
scourging
scowl
scramble
scrambled
scrambling
scrap
scrape
scraped
scrapie
scraping
scrapped
scrapping
scratch
scratches
scrawny
scream
screen
'screening'
screw
scrofula
scrotal
scrotum
scrub
scrubbed
scrubbing
scruple
scrupulous
scrutinize
scrutinized
scrutinizing
scrutiny
scurvy
scybala
scybalous
scybalum
seam

sear
search
searches
seasickness
season
seasonable
seasonal
seasonally
seat
sebaceous
seborrhoea
seborrhoeic
sebum
Secadrex®
secede
seceded
seceding
secession
secluded
seclusion
Seconal®
second
secondary
second-hand
secrecy
secret
secretagogue
secretarial
secretaries
secretary
secrete
secreted
secretin
secreting
secretion
secretive
secretor
secretory
sect
section
sector
Sectral®

secular
secure
secured
securing
securities
security
sedation
sedative
sedentary
sediment
see
seed
seedling
seeing
seek
seeking
seem
seemingly
seen
seep
seepage
seethe
seethed
seething
segment
segmental
segmentation
segregate
segregated
segregating
segregation
seize
seized
seizing
seizure
seldom
select
selection
selective
selector
selegiline
selenium

self
selfish
sell
sella turcica
selling
Sellotape®
Selsun®
selves
semantics
semblance
semen
semicircular canal
semicoma
semicomatose
semiconductor
semiconscious
semilunar
semimembranosus
  muscle
seminal
seminar
seminiferous
seminiferous tubule
seminoma
seminomata
semipermeable
semiprone
semispinalis muscle
Semitard MC®
semitendinosus
senate
senator
send
sending
senescence
senescent
Sengstaken tube
senile
senilis
senility
senior
seniority

Ss

senna
Senokot®
sensation
sense
sensed
senseless
sensibility
sensible
sensibly
sensing
sensitive
sensitivity
sensitization
sensitize
sensitizer
sensorineural
sensory
sent
sentence
sentenced
sentencing
sentiment
separate
separated
separating
separation
sepsis
septa
septal
septate
September
septic
septicaemia
septicaemic
septostomy
Septrin®
septuagenarian
septum
sequel
sequela
sequelae
sequence

sequential
sequester
sequestra
sequestrum
sera
Serc®
serial
series
serine
serious
serological
serologically
serology
seromucous
seropositive
serosa
serosal
serosanguineous
serotonin
serous
serpiginous
serrated
serration
serratus muscle
Sertoli's cell
serum
servant
serve
served
service
serviceable
serving
sesamoid
sessile
session
set
setting
settle
settled
settling
seven
seventeen

seventeenth
seventh
seventieth
seventy
sever
several
severance
severe
severed
severely
severing
severity
sew
sewage
sewed
sewer
sewing
sewn
sex
sexagenarian
sex-linked
sexual
sexuality
sexually
shadow
shaft
shake
shaken
shakily
shaking
shaky
shall
shallow
shame
shameful
shamefully
shampoo
shampooed
shampooing
shape
shaped
shaping

share
shared
sharing
sharp
sharpen
shatter
shave
shaved
shaving
sheaf
shear
sheared
shearing
sheath
sheaves
Sheehan's syndrome
sheepskin
sheer
sheet
Sheldon's body types
shelf
shell
shelter
shelve
shelves
shied
shield
shier
shiest
shift
Shigella
Shigella flexneri
Shigella sonnei
shilling
shimmer
shin
shine
shingles
shining
shiny
shiver
shock

shocking
shod
shoddily
shoddy
shoe
shoeing
shone
shook
shoot
shooting
shop
shopped
shopper
shopping
shorn
short
shortage
shortcoming
shorten
shorthand
shortly
short-time
shot
should
shoulder
shout
shove
shoved
shovel
shovelled
shovelling
shoving
show
showed
shower
showery
showing
shown
shrank
shrapnel
shred
shredded

shredding
shrewd
shriek
shrill
shrilly
shrink
shrinking
shrivel
shrivelled
shrivelling
shrug
shrugged
shrugging
shrunk
shrunken
shudder
shuffle
shuffled
shuffling
shun
shunned
shunning
shut
shutter
shutting
shuttle
shy
shyer
shyest
shying
shyly
shyness
sialagogue
sialogram
sialograph
sialographic
sialographically
sialography
sialolith
sib
sibling
sick

sicken
sickle-cell anaemia
sickling
sickly
sickness
side
sided
side-effect
siderosis
sideways
siding
sieve
sieved
sieving
sift
sigh
sight
sightseeing
sigmoid
sigmoidoscope
sigmoidoscopic
sigmoidoscopy
sign
signal
signalled
signalling
signatories
signatory
signature
significance
significant
signified
signify
signifying
Silastic®
silence
silenced
silencing
silent
silicon
silicone
silicosis

silk
silver
silver nitrate
similar
similarities
similarity
simple
Simplene®
simplicity
simplification
simplified
simplify
simplifying
simply
Sim's speculum
simulate
simulated
simulating
simulation
simulator
simultaneous
since
sincere
sincerely
sincerity
Sinemet®
Sinequan®
sine qua non
sinew
sing
singe
singed
singeing
singing
single
singled
singling
singly
singular
singularity
sink
sinking

Sino-atrial node
Sinu-atrial node
sinuous
sinus
sinuses
sinusitis
sinusoid
sinusoidal
sip
siphon
sipped
sipping
sister
sister-in-law
sisters-in-law
sit
site
sited
siting
sitting
situated
situation
sitz-bath
six
sixteen
sixteenth
sixth
sixtieth
sixty
sizable
size
sizeable
sized
sizing
Sjögren syndrome
skeletal
skeleton
skid
skidded
skidding
skies
skilful

skilfully
skill
skilled
skim
skimmed
skimming
skin
skinned
skinning
skinny
skull
sky
skylight
slack
slacken
slain
slam
slammed
slamming
slander
slanderous
slap
slapped
slapping
slash
slashes
slaughter
slave
slaver
slavery
slay
slaying
sledge
sledged
sledging
sleep
sleeper
sleepily
sleeping
sleeping sickness
sleepy
slender

slept
slew
slice
sliced
slicing
slid
slide
sliding
slight
slightly
slim
slimmed
slimming
slimy
sling
slinging
slip
slipped
slipped epiphysis
slippery
slipping
slit
slither
slitting
sliver
slobber
slogan
slop
slope
sloped
Slo-Phyllin®
sloping
slopped
slopping
slot
slotted
slotting
slouch
slough
sloughed
sloughing
slow

Slow-K®
slow release
Slow-Trasicor®
slow virus
sludge
sluggish
sluice
slum
slumber
slung
slur
slurred
slurring
slush
slushy
smack
small
small-for-dates
smallness
smallpox
smart
smash
smashes
smattering
smear
smeared
smegma
smell
smelled
smelling
smelly
smelt
smelted
smelting
smile
smiled
smiling
smirk
smithereens
Smith-Petersen nail
smog
smoke

smoked
smokeless
smoker
smoking
smoky
smooth
smother
smoulder
smudge
smudged
smudging
snack
snake
snaked
snaking
snap
snapped
snapping
snatch
snatches
sneaky
sneeze
sneezed
sneezing
Snellen's test types
sniff
snip
snipped
snipping
snobbery
snobbish
snooze
snoozed
snoozing
snore
snored
snoring
snout
snow
snub
snubbed
snubbing

snuffbox
snuffles
soak
so-and-so
soap
soapiness
soapy
soar
sob
sobbed
sobbing
sober
sobriety
sociability
sociable
sociably
social
socialization
socially
socioeconomic
sociological
sociology
socket
soda
sodden
sodium
sodomy
Sofradex®
Soframycin®
Sofra-Tulle®
soften
softener
software
soggy
soil
solar
solarium
solar plexus
sold
solder
soldier
sole

soleal
solemn
solemnity
solemnly
solenoid
soleus muscle
solicit
solicitor
solicitous
solid
solidarity
solidified
solidify
solidifying
solidity
solitary
solitude
Soliwax®
Solpadeine®
solubility
soluble
solute
solution
solve
solved
solvent
solving
soma
somatic
somatization
somatology
Somatonorm 4IU®
somatostatin
somatotrophic
somatotrophin
somatrem
sombre
some
somebody
someone
somersault
something

somnambulation
somnambulism
somnambulist
Somogyi unit
Soneryl®
sonic
Sonicaid®
son-in-law
Sonne dysentery
sonograph
sonometer
sons-in-law
soon
sooner
soothe
soothed
soothing
sophisticated
sophistication
soporific
Sorbichew®
sorbitol
sore
soreness
sorrow
sorry
sort
sortie
Sotacor®
sotalol
Sotazide®
souffle
sought
sound
source
southern
Souttar's tube
sovereign
sow
sowed
sowing
sown

soya
soya bean
spa
space
spaced
spacing
spacious
spade
Spalding's sign
span
Spanish
spanned
spanning
spansule
spare
spared
Sparine®
sparing
sparingly
spark
sparkle
sparkled
sparkling
sparse
spasm
spasmodic
spasmodically
spastic
spasticity
spat
spate
spatula
spay
speak
speaking
spear
special
specialist
specialities
speciality
specialization
specialize

specialized
specializing
specially
specialties
specialty
species
specific
specifically
specification
specificity
specified
specify
specifying
specimen
speck
spectacles
spectator
spectinomycin
spectograph
spectra
spectrograph
spectrometer
spectrometry
spectrophotometer
spectrophotometric
spectrophotometry
spectroscope
spectroscopic
spectrum
spectrums
specula
speculate
speculated
speculating
speculation
speculative
speculum
sped
speech
speeches
speechless
speed

speeded
spell
spelled
spelling
spelt
spend
spending
spent
sperm
spermatic
spermatocele
spermatocyte
spermatogenesis
spermatogonium
spermatozoa
spermatozoon
spermicidal
spermicide
spew
sphenoid
sphenoidal
sphenopalatine
sphere
spherical
spherocyte
spherocytic
spherocytosis
sphincter
sphincteric
sphincterotomy
sphingomyelin
sphingomyelinase
sphygmomanometer
sphygmomanometry
spica
spice
spiciness
spicule
spicy
spider
Spigelian hernia
spigot

spiked
spiky
spill
spillage
spilled
spilling
spilt
spin
spina
spina bifida
spina bifida occulta
spinal
spinal cord
spinalis
spine
Spinhaler®
Spinhaler insufflator®
spinning
spinocerebellar
spinothalamic
spinous
spiral
spiralled
spiralling
spirilla
Spirillum
spirit
spirochaetal
spirochaete
spirograph
spirographic
spirography
spirometer
spirometric
spirometry
spironolactone
spit
spite
spiteful
spitefully
spitting
spittle

Spitz-Holter valve
splanchnic
splash
splashes
splay
splay-footed
spleen
splendid
splendour
splenectomize
splenectomy
splenic
spleniculus
splenium
splenius
splenization
splenomegaly
splenorenal
splint
splinter
split
splitting
spoil
spoiled
spoiling
spoilt
spoke
spoken
spokesman
spondylitic
spondylitis
spondylolisthesis
spondylolisthetic
spondylosis
sponge
sponged
spongiform
sponging
spongiosa
spongiose
spongiosis
spongy

sponsor
spontaneity
spontaneous
spoon
spoonful
sporadic
sporadically
spore
sporicidal
Sporozoa
sport
sporting
sportsman
sportsmen
sporulation
spot
spotless
spotted
spotted fever
spotting
spotty
spouse
sprain
sprained
spraining
sprang
spray
spread
spread-eagled
spreading
sprightlily
sprightly
spring
springing
sprinkle
sprinkled
sprinkler
sprinkling
sprue
sprung
spun
spur

spurious
spurious diarrhoea
spurred
spurring
sputum
squabble
squabbled
squabbling
squad
squadron
squalor
squamous
squander
square
squash
squat
squatted
squatting
squeak
squeal
squeamish
squeeze
squeezed
squeezing
squint
squirm
squirt
stab
stabbed
stabbing
stability
stabilize
stabilized
stabilizer
stabilizing
stable
staccato
staff
stage
staged
stagger
staggered

staggering
staging
stagnant
stagnate
stagnated
stagnating
stain
stainless
staircase
stale
stall
stallion
stalwart
stamina
stammer
stammered
stammering
stance
stanch
stand
standard
standardization
standardize
standardized
standardizing
standby
stand-in
standing
standstill
stank
stanozolol
stapedectomy
stapedial
stapediolysis
stapedius
stapes
staphylococcal
Staphylococcus
staple
starch
starches
starchy

stare
stared
staring
start
startle
startled
startling
starvation
starve
starved
starving
stasis
state
stated
statement
static
stating
station
stationary
stationer
stationery
statistical
statistically
statistician
statistics
status
status asthmaticus
status epilepticus
status quo
statutory
staunch
stave
staved
staving
stay
Staycept®
steadied
steadily
steady
steadying
steaglate
steal

stealing
steatorrhoea
steel
steely
steep
steer
Stein-Leventhal
  syndrome
Stelazine®
stellate
stem
Stemetil®
stemmed
stemming
stench
stenosed
stenoses
stenosis
stenotic
step
stepmother
stepped
stepping
stercobilin
stercobilinogen
stercoporphyrin
sterculia
stereo
stereognosis
stereognostic
stereophonic
stereoscopic
stereotactic
stereotaxy
stereotype
stereotyped
sterile
sterility
sterilization
sterilize
sterilized
sterilizer

sterilizing
Steri-Strip®
stern
sternal
sternoclavicular
sternocleidomastoid
sternocostal
sternotomy
sternum
steroid
steroidogenesis
stertor
stertorous
stet
stethoscope
stethoscopic
Stevens-Johnson
  syndrome
stick
sticking
sticky
sties
stiff
stiffen
stifle
stifled
stifling
stigmata
stigmatization
stilboestrol
stilette
still
stillbirth
stillborn
stillness
Still's disease
stimulant
stimulate
stimulated
stimulating
stimulator
stimuli

stimulus
sting
stinging
stink
stinking
stipulate
stipulated
stipulating
stipulation
stir
stirred
stirring
stirrup
stitch
stitches
stock
stockinette
stoicism
Stokes-Adams
  syndrome
stole
stolen
stoma
stomach
Stomahesive®
stomal
stomata
stomatitis
stone
stood
stool
stoop
stop
stoppage
stopped
stopper
stopping
storage
store
stored
storey
stories

storing
story
stout
stoutness
stove
stove-in chest
strabismus
straddle
straddled
straddling
straight
straighten
straightness
strain
strainer
straitjacket
strand
strange
strangeness
stranger
strangle
strangled
strangling
strangulated
strangulation
strangury
strap
strapped
strapping
strata
stratagem
strategic
strategically
strategies
strategist
strategy
stratification
stratified
stratum
stratum corneum
stratus
straw

strawberry tongue
stream
streamline
streamlined
streamlining
street
strength
strengthen
strenuous
streptococcal
Streptococcus
Streptococcus faecalis
Streptococcus
  pneumoniae
Streptococcus
  pyogenes
streptodornase
streptokinase
streptolysin
Streptomyces
streptomycin
stress
stresses
stretch
stretcher
stretches
strew
strewed
strewing
strewn
stria
striae
striate
striated
stricken
strict
stricture
stride
striding
stridor
stridulous
strike

striking
string
stringencies
stringency
stringent
stringing
strip
striped
stripped
stripping
stripy
strive
striven
striving
stroboscope
stroboscopic
strode
stroke
stroked
stroking
stroma
stromal
Stromba®
strongyliasis
Strongyloides
Strongyloides
  stercoralis
strongyloidiasis
Strongylus
strontium
strontium-90
strove
struck
structural
structurally
structure
structured
struggle
struggled
struggling
strung
strychnine

Stryker bed
stub
stubbed
stubbing
stubborn
stubbornness
stubby
stuck
student
studied
studies
studio
studious
study
studying
stuff
stuffy
Stugeron®
stumble
stumbled
stumbling
stump
stun
stung
stunk
stunned
stunning
stunt
stunted
stupid
stupidity
stupor
stuporous
sturdily
sturdiness
sturdy
Sturge-Weber
  syndrome
stutter
stuttering
St Vitus' dance
sty

stye
styes
style
styled
styling
stylish
styloglossal
styloglossus
stylohyoid
styloid
stylomastoid
subacromial
subacute
subarachnoid
subcapital
subclavian
subclinical
subcommittee
subconjunctival
subconjunctivally
subconscious
subcostal
subculture
subcutaneous
subcutaneously
subcuticular
subdue
subdued
subduing
subdural
subendocardial
subfertility
subject
subjective
subjectiveness
subjectivity
sublimate
sublimation
sublime
subliminal
sublingual
subluxation

submandibular
submerge
submerged
submerging
submersion
submission
submit
submitted
submitting
submucosa
submucosal
submucous
subnormal
subnormality
subordinate
subordinated
subordinating
subperiosteal
subphrenic
subscribe
subscribed
subscribing
subscription
subsequent
subside
subsided
subsidiaries
subsidiary
subsidies
subsiding
subsidize
subsidized
subsidizing
subsidy
sub-species
substance
substantia
substantial
substantially
substantiate
substantiated
substantiating

substitute
substituted
substituting
substitution
substrate
subtotal
subtract
subungual
suburban
succedaneum
succeed
success
successes
successful
successfully
succession
successive
successor
succinate
succinct
succinylcholine
succumb
succussion
suckle
suckled
suckling
sucralfate
sucrose
suction
Sudafed®
sudden
suddenly
suddenness
Sudeck's atrophy
sue
sued
suffer
suffice
sufficed
sufficient
sufficing
suffocate

suffocated
suffocating
suffocation
suffusion
sugar
sugary
suggest
suggestibility
suggestible
suggestion
suggestive
suicidal
suicide
suing
suit
suitability
suitable
suitably
suitcase
suite
sulci
sulconazole
sulcus
sulfadoxine
sulfametopyrazine
sulindac
sullenness
sulphacetamide
sulphadiazine
sulphadimethoxine
sulphadimidine
sulpha drugs
sulphaguanidine
sulphaloxate
sulphamethoxazole
sulphasalazine
sulphate
sulphaurea
sulphide
sulphinpyrazone
sulphonamide
sulphonylurea

Ss

sulphonylureas
sulphur
sulphur dioxide
sulphuric
sulpiride
Sultrin®
sum
summaries
summarily
summarize
summarized
summarizing
summary
summation
summed
summing
summon
summoned
summoning
sunburn
sunburned
sunburnt
Sunday
sundries
sundry
sunflower
sung
sunk
sunken
sunnily
sunny
sunscreen
sunstroke
superannuated
superannuation
superb
superego
superfemale
superficial
superficialis
superficially
superfluous

superinfection
superintendent
superior
superiority
superiorly
superlative
supernatant
supernumerary
superolateral
superomedial
supersede
superseded
superseding
supersensitive
superstition
superstitious
supervise
supervised
supervising
supervision
supervisor
supinate
supinator
supine
supple
supplement
supplementary
suppleness
supplied
supplies
supply
supplying
support
supporter
suppose
supposed
supposedly
supposing
supposition
suppository
suppress
suppressant

suppression
suppressor
suppurate
suppurated
suppurating
suppuration
suppurative
supraclavicular
supracondylar
supranuclear
supraorbital
suprapubic
suprarenal
suprascapular
supraspinatus muscle
suprasternal
supratentorial
supraventricular
supremacy
supreme
sural
suramin
surcharge
sure
surely
surface
surfaced
surfacing
surfactant
surfeit
Surgam®
surge
surged
surgeon
surgeries
surgery
surgical
surgically
surging
Surmontil®
surname
surpass

surplus
surprise
surprised
surprising
surrender
surrogate
surround
surroundings
surveillance
survey
surveyor
survival
survive
survived
surviving
survivor
Suscard®
susceptibility
susceptible
suspect
suspend
suspension
suspensory
suspicion
suspicious
Sustac®
sustain
sustenance
suture
suxamethonium
swab
swabbed
swabbing
swaddle
swaddled
swaddling
swallow
swam
swamp
Swan-Ganz catheter
swap
swapped

swapping
swarm
swear
swearing
sweat
sweated
sweating
sweaty
Swedish
sweep
sweeping
sweeten
sweetener
swell
swelled
swelling
Swenson's operation
swept
swerve
swerved
swerving
swift
swim
swimmer
swimming
swing
swinging
Swiss
switch
switchboard
switches
swollen
swop
swopped
swopping
swore
sworn
swum
swung
sycosis barbae
Sydenham's chorea
syllabi

syllabize
syllable
syllabus
syllabuses
symbiosis
symbiotic
symbol
symbolic
symbolically
symbolize
symbolized
symbolizing
Symmetrel®
symmetrical
symmetrically
symmetry
sympathectomy
sympathetic
sympathetically
sympathize
sympathized
sympathizing
sympathomimetic
sympathy
symphyseal
symphysis
symposium
symposiums
symptom
symptomatic
symptomatology
Synacthen®
Synalar®
synapse
synapsis
synchronize
synchronized
synchronizing
syncope
syncytial
syncytium
syndactyly

syndesmophyte
syndicate
syndrome
synechia
synechiae
synergic
synergism
synergist
synergistic
synergy
synonym
synopses
synopsis
synostosis
synovectomy
synovial
synovitis
synovium
Synphase®
Syntaris®
syntax
synthesis
synthesize
synthetase
synthetic
synthetically
synthetize
Syntocinon®
Syntometrine®
syphilide
syphilis
syphilitic
syringe
syringobulbia
syringomyelia
syrup
system
systematic
systematically
systematization
systematize
systemic

systole
systolic

Tt

tabes
tabetic
table
tableau
tableaux
tabled
tablespoonful
tablet
tabling
tabloid
taboo
tabulate
tabulated
tabulating
tache
tachyarrhythmia
tachycardia
tachypnoea
tachypnoeic
tacit
taciturn
tack
tackle
tackled
tackling
tact
tactful
tactfully
tactical
tactically
tactician

tactics
tactile
tactless
tadpole
Taenia
Taenia echinococcus
Taenia saginata
Taenia solium
taenicide
Tagamet®
tail
tailor
taint
take
taken
takeover
taking
talampicillin
talc
talcum (powder)
tale
talent
talented
talipes
talisman
talkative
tall
tallied
tallies
tallness
tally
tallying
talon
talus
tambourine
tame
tamed
taming
tamoxifen
tamper
tampon
tamponade

Tt

Tampovagan
  Stilboestrol and
  Lactic Acid
tan
tandem
tang
tangent
tangerine
tangible
tangibly
tangle
tangled
tangling
tankard
tanker
tanned
tanneries
tannery
tannic acid
tannin
tanning
tantamount to
tantrum
tap
tape
taped
tapestries
tapestry
tapetum
tapeworm
taping
tapioca
tapped
tapping
tarantula
Tarcortin®
tardily
tardive
tardive dyskinesia
tardy
tare
target

tariff
tarpaulin
tarsal
tarsalgia
tarsometatarsal
tarsoplasty
tarsorrhaphy
tarsus
tart
tartar
tartrate
Tartrazine
task
tasselled
taste
tasted
tasteful
tastefully
tasteless
tasting
tasty
tattered
tatters
tattoo
taught
taunt
taurine
taurocholate
taut
tauten
Tavegil®
taxable
taxation
taxi
taxidermist
taxidermy
taxied
taxiing
taxis
Tay-Sachs' disease
teach
teacher

teaching
teak
team
teapot
tear
tearing
tease
teased
teasing
teaspoonful
teat
technetium
technical
technicalities
technicality
technically
technician
technique
technological
technologically
technologies
technologist
technology
tectum
teddy-bear
tedious
tedium
tee
teed
teeing
teem
teenage
teenager
teens
teeth
teethe
teethed
teething
teetotal
teetotaller
tegmen
tegmentum

Tegretol®
tela
telangiectasia
telangiectasis
telangiectatic
telegram
telegraph
telegraphic
telemetry
telencephalon
telepathic
telepathically
telepathy
telephone
telephoned
telephoning
telephonist
telephoto lens
telescope
telescoped
telescopic
telescopically
telescoping
teletext
televise
televised
televising
television
telex
tell
teller
telling
telogen
telophase
temazepam
temerity
Temgesic®
temper
temperament
temperamental
temperamentally
temperance

temperate
temperature
tempest
tempestuous
template
temple
temporal
temporary
temporomandibular
temporoparietal
tempt
temptation
tempting
Tempulin®
tenable
tenacious
tenacity
tenaculum
tenancies
tenancy
tenant
tendencies
tendency
tender
tendinous
tendon
tendonitis
tendril
tenectomy
tenesmus
tenet
tennis
tennis elbow
tenon
Tenoret-50®
Tenoretic®
Tenormin®
tenosynovitis
tenotomy
tense
Tensilon®
tension

tensor
tensor fasciae latae
tensor palati
tensor tympani
tentacle
tentative
tenterhooks
tentorial
tentorium
Tenuate Dospan®
tenuous
tenure
tepid
teratogen
teratogenesis
teratogenic
teratogenicity
teratological
teratologically
teratology
teratoma
teratomata
teratomatous
terazosin
terbutaline
tercentenary
teres
terfenadine
terlipressin
terminal
terminate
terminated
terminating
termination
termini
terminology
terminus
terminuses
termite
terodiline
Terolin®
terpene

terrace
terracing
Terra-Cortril®
terracotta
terra firma
terrain
terrestrial
terrible
terribly
terrific
terrifically
terrified
terrify
terrifying
territorial
territories
territory
terror
terrorism
terrorist
tertian
tertiary
testament
testes
testicle
testicular
testified
testify
testifying
testily
testimonial
testimonies
testimony
testis
testosterone
test-tube baby
test-types
testy
tetanus
tetany
tête-à-tête
tetrabenazine

tetrachlorethylene
tetracosactrin
tetracycline
tetradecyl
Tetralogy of Fallot
tetraplegia
tetraplegic
text
textile
textual
texture
thalami
thalamic
thalamotomy
thalamus
thalassaemia
thalidomide
thankful
thankfully
thankless
thanksgiving
thaw
theatre
theatrical
theatrically
theca
thecal
theft
their
theirs
them
theme
themselves
thenar
theologian
theological
theology
theophylline
theorem
theoretical
theoretically
theories

theorize
theorized
theorizing
theory
therapeutic
therapeutically
therapeutics
therapist
therapy
there
thereabouts
therefore
therm
thermal
thermogenesis
thermography
thermometer
thermophilic
thermoreceptor
thermoregulation
thermoresistant
Thermos® (flask)
thermostat
thesaurus
theses
thesis
they'd
they'll
they're
thiabendazole
thiamine
thiazide
thick
thicken
thickness
thicknesses
thief
thiethylperazine
thieves
thievish
thigh
thimble

thin
thing
think
thinking
thinned
thinner
thinness
thinnest
thinning
thiocyanate
thioguanine
thiopentone
thioridazine
thiosulphate
thiotepa
thiouracil
thioxanthene
third
third-rate
thirst
thirstily
thirsty
thirteen
thirteenth
thirtieth
thirty
thistle
thong
thoracic
thoracocentesis
thoracolumbar
thoracoplasty
thoracotomy
thorax
thorn
thorny
thorough
thoroughfare
thoroughgoing
though
thought
thoughtful

thoughtfully
thoughtfulness
thoughtless
thousand
thousandth
Thovaline®
thrall
thread
threadbare
threadworm
threadworn
threat
threaten
threatened
threatened abortion
threatening
thresh
threshold
threw
thrift
thriftily
thrifty
thrill
thriller
thrilling
thrive
thrived
thriving
throat
throb
throbbed
throbbing
throes
thrombectomy
thrombi
thrombin
thrombo-angiitis
thrombo-arteritis
thrombocyte
thrombocythaemia
thrombocytopenia
thrombocytopenic

thrombocytopenic
 purpura
thrombocytosis
thrombo-embolic
thrombo-embolism
thrombo-endarter·
 ectomy
thrombo-endarteritis
thrombogen
thrombogenesis
thrombogenic
thrombolysis
thrombolytic
thrombophlebitic
thrombophlebitis
thromboplastin
thromboses
thrombosis
thrombotic
thrombus
throne
throng
throttle
throttled
throttling
through
throughout
throughput
throw
throwback
throwing
thrown
thrush
thrushes
thrust
thrusting
thud
thudded
thudding
thumb
thunder
thunderstruck

Thursday
thus
thwart
thyme
thymectomy
thymidine
thymine
thymol
thymoma
thymomata
thymoxamine
thymus
thyroglossal
thyroid
thyroidectomy
thyroiditis
thyrotoxic
thyrotoxicosis
thyrotrophic
thyrotrophin-releasing
thyroxine
tiaprofenic acid
tibia
tibial
tibialis
tibiofemoral
tibiofibular
tic
ticarcillin
tic douloureux
tick
ticket
tickle
tickled
tickling
ticklish
tickly
tidal
tide
tidied
tidier
tidiest

tidily
tidiness
tidings
tidy
tidying
tie
tied
tier
Tigason®
tight
tighten
tightened
tightening
tightness
tights
tile
tiled
tiling
till
timber
timbre
time
timed
timeless
timely
timer
timetable
timid
timidity
timing
Timodine®
timolol
Timoptol®
timorous
tincture
Tinea
Tinea capitis
Tinea corporis
Tinea cruris
Tineafax®
Tinea pedis
Tine test

tinfoil
tinge
tinged
tinging
tingle
tingled
tingling
tinidazole
tinnitus
tint
tiny
tioconazole
tip
tipped
tipping
tiptoe
tiptoed
tiptoeing
tirade
tire
tired
tireless
tiresome
tiring
tissue
titanium
title
titled
titrate
titration
titre
titubation
titular
toad
toadstool
toast
toaster
tobacco
tobacco amblyopia
tobacconist
toboggan
tobramycin

tocainide
tocograph
tocography
tocopherol
tocopheryl
tocopheryl acetate
tocopheryl succinate
today
toddler
Todd's paralysis
toddy
toffee
Tofranil®
together
toilet
token
tolazamide
tolbutamide
told
tolerable
tolerably
tolerance
tolerate
tolerated
tolerating
toleration
toll
tolmetin
tolnaftate
tomato
tomatoes
tomb
tomboy
tombstone
tome
tomogram
tomograph
tomographic
tomographically
tomography
tomorrow
ton

tone
toned
tongs
tongue
tongue-tie
tongue-tied
tonic
tonic-clonic
tonicity
tonight
toning
tonnage
tonne
tonography
tonometer
tonometry
tonsil
tonsilitis
tonsillar
tonsillectomy
tonsillitis
tonsils
tonus
took
tool
tooth
tooth-ache
Topal®
tophaceous
tophi
tophus
topic
topical
topically
Topicycline®
Topilar®
topographical
topographically
topography
torch
torches
tore

Tories
torment
torn
tornado
tornadoes
torpedo
torpedoed
torpedoes
torpedoing
torque
torrent
torrential
torsion
torso
torsos
torticollis
tortoise
tortuous
torture
tortured
torturing
torulopsosis
Tory
toss
total
totalled
totalling
totally
totipotence
totipotent
touch
touchily
touchiness
touching
touchy
tough
toughen
toupee
tour
Tourette's syndrome
tourism
tourist

tournament
tourniquet
tousled
tow
toward
towards
towel
towelled
towelling
tower
town
toxaemia
toxaemic
toxic
toxicity
toxicology
toxicosis
toxin
Toxocara
toxocariasis
toxoid
Toxoplasma
Toxoplasma gondii
toxoplasmosis
trabecula
trabeculae
trabecular
trabeculation
trabeculotomy
trace
traceable
traced
trace element
tracer
trachea
tracheal
tracheitis
tracheobronchial
tracheobronchitis
tracheo-oesophageal
tracheostomy
tracheotomy

trachoma
trachomatous
tracing
track
tract
traction
tractor
tractotomy
tractus
trade
traded
trade-in
trademark
tradename
trader
tradesman
trade union
trading
tradition
traditional
traditionally
traffic
trafficked
trafficking
tragedies
tragedy
tragi
tragic
tragically
tragus
trainee
trait
traitor
traitorous
tramp
trample
trampled
trampling
trampoline
trance
tranexamic acid
tranquil

tranquillity
tranquillizer
tranquilly
transabdominal
transabdominally
transaction
transaminases
transatlantic
transcend
transcriptase
transcription
transcutaneous
transducer
transection
transfer
transferable
transference
transferred
transferring
transfiguration
transfix
transform
transformation
transformer
transfuse
transfusion
Transiderm-Nitro®
transience
transient
transient ischaemic
    attack (TIA)
transillumination
transistor
transit
transition
transitional
transitorily
transitory
translate
translated
translating
translation

Tt

translator
Translet®
translocation
translucence
translucency
translucent
transmigration
transmissibility
transmissible
transmission
transmit
transmitted
transmitter
transmitting
transmural
transmutation
transparencies
transparency
transparent
transplacental
transplacentally
transplant
transplantation
transport
transportation
transpose
transposed
transposing
transposition
trans-sexual
trans-sexualism
trans-sphenoidal
transudate
transudation
transurethral
  prostatectomy
transverse
transversus abdominis
transvesical
transvesical
  prostatectomy
transvestite

transvestitism
tranylcypromine
trap
trapezium
trapezius
trapezoid
trapped
trapping
trappings
Trasicor®
Trasidrex®
trauma
traumatic
traumatological
traumatology
travel
travelled
traveller
traveller's cheque
travelling
Travogyn®
trawler
Traxam®
trazodone
treacherous
treachery
treacle
tread
treason
treasonable
treasure
treasurer
treasure-trove
treasuries
treasury
treat
treaties
treatise
treatment
treaty
treble
trek

trekked
trekking
Trematoda
trematode
tremble
trembled
trembling
tremendous
tremor
tremulous
trenchant
trench foot
Trendelenburg's
  operation
Trendelenburg's sign
trendy
treosulfan
trephine
trepidation
Treponema
Treponema pallidum
trespass
trespasses
trestle
tretinoin
triad
Tri-Adcortyl®
trial
triamcinolone
triamterene
triangle
triangular
triazolam
tribal
tribe
tribulation
tribunal
tribune
tributaries
tributary
tribute
triceps

trichiasis
Trichinella
trichinellosis
trichiniasis
trichinosis
trichloracetic acid
trichloroethylene
trichomonacide
trichomonad
trichomonal
Trichomonas
Trichomonas vaginalis
trichomoniasis
Trichophyton
Trichophyton rubrum
Trichosporon
Trichostrongylus
Trichuris
trickery
trickle
trickled
trickling
triclofos
triclosan
tricolour
tricuspid
tricycle
tricyclic
tried
tries
trifle
trifled
trifling
trifluoperazine
trifluperidol
trigeminal
trigeminal neuralgia
trigger
triggered
trigger finger
triggering
triglyceride

trigonal
trigone
trigonitis
trigonometry
triiodothyronine
trilogies
trilogy
trilostane
Triludan®
trim
trimeprazine
trimester
trimetaphan
  camsylate
trimethoprim
trimipramine
trimmed
trimming
Trimovate®
trinitrate
trinket
Trinordiol®
TriNovum®
trio
trios
trip
tripe
triple
triplet
triplicate
triploid
Triplopen®
tripod
tripotassium
  dicitratobismuthate
tripped
tripping
triprolidine
Triptafen®
Trisequens®
trisilicate
trismus

trisodium edetate
trisomy
trisomy 21
tritiated
tritium
triumph
triumphant
trivial
trivialities
triviality
trocar
trochanter
trochanteric
trochlea
trochlear
Trochostrongylus
trod
trodden
Troisier's ganglion or
  sign
trolley
trooper
trophic
trophies
trophoblast
trophoblastic
trophy
tropic
tropical
tropicamide
Trosyl®
trouble
troubled
troublesome
troubling
Trousseau's sign
trousers
truancy
truant
truce
truculent
true

Tt

truffle
truly
trumpet
truncal
truncate
truncated
truncus
trunk
truss
trusses
trust
trustee
trustful
trustfully
trustworthy
truth
truthful
truthfully
truthfulness
try
trying
trypanocide
Trypanosoma
trypanosomiasis
trypsin
trypsinogen
Tryptizol®
tryptophan
trysinogen
tsetse fly
tubal
tubby
tube
Tubegauz®
tuber
tubercle
tubercular
tuberculin
tuberculoma
tuberculosis
tuberculostatic
tuberculous

tuberosity
tuberous sclerosis
Tubigrip®
tubing
tubocurarine
tubo-overian
tubular
tubular necrosis
tubular stockinette
tubule
Tuesday
Tuinal®
tuition
tularaemia
tulip
tulle
tulle gras
tumble
tumbled
tumbler
tumbling
tumescence
tummies
tummy
tumor
tumour
tumult
tumultuous
tune
tuned
tuneful
tunefully
tuneless
tunic
tunica
tunica albuginea
tunica intima
tunica media
tunica vaginalis
tuning
tunnel
tunnelled

tunnelling
turban
turbid
turbidity
turbinate
turbine
turbinectomy
turbulence
turbulent
tureen
turgid
turkey
Turkish
turmoil
Turner syndrome
turnstile
turntable
turpentine
turpentine liniment
turquoise
turtleneck
tussle
tutor
tutorial
tweezers
twelfth
twelve
twentieth
twenty
twilight
twin
twinge
twist
twitch
twitches
twofold
tycoon
tying
Tylex®
tyloxapol
tympanic
tympanitis

tympanoplasty
tympanosclerosis
tympanum
type
typed
typewriter
typhoid
typhoon
typhus
typical
typically
typing
typist
tyramine
tyrannical
tyrannically
tyranny
tyre
tyrosine
tyrosinosis

Uu

ubiquitous
Ubretid®
uglier
ugliest
ugliness
ugly
ulcer
ulcerate
ulceration
ulcerative
ulcerative colitis
ulcerogenic
ulcerous
ulna
ulnar

ulterior
ultimata
ultimate
ultimately
ultimatum
ultimatums
Ultrabase®
ultracentrifuge
ultrafiltration
ultrasonic
ultrasonographically
ultrasonography
ultrasound
Ultratard®
ultraviolet
umbilical
umbilicated
umbilicus
unable
unaccountable
unaccountably
unadulterated
unanimity
unanimous
unapproachable
unaware
unawares
unbalanced
unbend
unbending
unbent
uncared for
uncertain
uncharted
uncle
uncoil
uncommon
unconscious
unconsciously
unconsciousness
uncus
undecenoate

undeniable
undeniably
underclothes
undercover
undercurrent
undercut
undercutting
underdeveloped
underdone
underestimate
underestimated
underestimating
underexposure
undergo
undergoing
undergone
underground
underhand
underline
underlined
underlining
underlying
undermine
undermined
undermining
underneath
under-penetration
underprivileged
underrate
underrated
underrating
undersigned
understand
understandable
understandably
understanding
understatement
understood
undertake
undertaken
undertaking
undertook

Uu

underwear
underwent
undid
undifferentiation
undo
undoing
undone
undoubted
undress
undue
undulent
unduly
uneasily
uneasy
unemployed
unemployment
unequal
unequalled
unequivocal
unequivocally
unerring
uneven
unexpected
unforgettable
unforgettably
unfortunate
unfortunately
unfounded
ungracious
ungrateful
ungratefully
ungual
unguarded
unguentum
Unguentum Merck®
unhappily
unhappiness
unhappy
unhealthily
unhealthy
unicellular
unification

unified
uniform
uniformity
unify
unifying
unilateral
unilaterally
uninterrupted
uniocular
union
uniovular
unipolar
unipotent
unique
uniquely
unit
unite
united
uniting
unity
universal
universally
universe
universities
university
unleash
unless
unlikely
unloose
unloosed
unloosing
unluckily
unlucky
unmentionable
unmistakable
unmistakably
unmitigated
unmoved
unnecessarily
unnecessary
unobtrusive
unpalatable

unparalleled
unpremeditated
unprepossessing
unpretentious
unprincipled
unravel
unravelled
unravelling
unremitting
unrivalled
unruly
unsaturated
unscathed
unscrew
unsophisticated
unsound
unspeakable
unspeakably
unstructured
unsuspecting
unthinkable
until
untimely
untoward
untrue
untruth
untruthful
untruthfully
unusual
unusually
unwieldy
unwitting
unwonted
unworthy
upbringing
upgrade
upgraded
upgrading
upheaval
upheld
uphold
upholding

upkeep
upland
upper
uppermost
upper respiratory tract
upright
upset
upsetting
upside-down
upstairs
upstanding
uptake
up-to-date
urachal
urachus
uraemia
uraemic
uranium
urate
urea
ureter
ureteral
ureteric
ureterolithotomy
ureterostomy
urethra
urethral
urethritis
urethrocele
urethrography
urethrotomy
urge
urged
urgency
urgent
urging
uric acid
uricosuric
urinalysis
urinary
urinary retention
urinate

urinated
urinating
urination
urine
uriniferous
Urispas®
urobilin
urobilinogen
urobilinuria
urodynamics
urofollitrophin
urogenital
urogram
urography
urokinase
urological
urologically
urologist
urology
uropathy
uroporphyrin
urostomy
urothelial
ursodeoxycholic acid
urticaria
urticarial
usable
usage
use
used
useful
usefully
usefulness
useless
using
usual
usually
utensil
uteri
uterine
uteroplacental
uterosacral

uterosalpingography
uterovaginal
uterovesical
uterus
utilities
utility
utilization
utilize
utilized
utilizing
utmost
utricle
utterly
uvea
uveal
uveitis
uvula

Vv

vacancies
vacancy
vacant
vacate
vacated
vacating
vacation
vaccinate
vaccinated
vaccinating
vaccination
vaccine
vaccinia
vaccinial
vacuolate
vacuolated
vacuum
vagal

Vv

vagi
vagina
vaginal
vaginismus
vaginitis
vagotomy
vague
vaguely
vagus nerve
valerate
valga
valgum
valgus
valid
validate
validity
valine
Valium®
Vallergan®
valproate
Valsalva manoeuvre
valuable
valuation
valuator
value
value-added tax
valued
valuing
valuole
valve
valvoplasty
valvotomy
valvular
valvulotomy
vancomycin
vandal
vandalism
Van den Bergh's test
vanguard
vanish
vanities
vanity

vanyl mandelic acid
vaporization
vaporize
vaporized
vaporizer
vaporizing
vapour
vara
variability
variable
variably
variance
variant
variation
Varicella
Varicella zoster
varicelliform
varices
varicocele
varicose
varicosity
Varidase®
varied
variegated
varieties
variety
Variola
variolate
various
varix
varum
varus
vary
varying
vas
vasa
vascular
vascularity
vascularization
vascularize
vasculature
vasculitis

vas deferens
vase
vasectomy
Vaseline®
vasoconstriction
vasoconstrictor
vasodilatation
vasodilator
vasomotor
vasopressin
vasopressor
vasospasm
vasovagal attack
vastus
Vater's ampulla
vector
vectorcardiogram
vectorcardiography
vecuronium
vegan
vegetable
vegetarian
vegetarianism
vegetate
vegetated
vegetating
vegetation
vegetative
vehement
vehicle
vehicular
vein
veined
veinography
velamentous
vellum
velocities
velocity
Velosulin®
velum
vena cava
vending

veneer
venepuncture
venereal
venereal disease
venereologist
venereology
venesection
venogram
venography
venom
venomous
venous
ventilate
ventilated
ventilating
ventilation
ventilator
ventilatory
Ventolin®
Ventouse extraction
ventral
ventrally
ventricle
ventricular
ventriculogram
ventriculography
ventriculostomy
ventrosuspension
venture
ventured
Venturi®
venturing
venue
venule
veracity
verapamil
verbatim
verbose
verdict
verdigris
verge
verged

verging
verification
verified
verify
verifying
vermiform
vermiform appendix
vermin
verminous
Vermox®
vernix caseosa
verruca
verrucae
versatile
versatility
version
versus
vertebra
vertebrae
vertebral
vertebrate
vertebrobasilar
  insufficiency (VBI)
vertex
vertical
vertically
vertices
vertiginous
vertigo
vesical
vesicle
vesicoureteric
vesicovaginal
vesicular
vessel
vestibular
vestibule
vestige
vestigial
vet
veteran
veterinary

veto
vetoed
vetoes
vetoing
vetted
vetting
viability
viable
vial
Vibramycin®
vibrant
vibrate
vibrated
vibrating
vibration
vibrator
vibratory
Vibrio cholerae
vibrissae
vicarious
vice versa
vicinity
vicious
vicissitude
victim
victimization
victories
victorious
victory
vidarabine
videotape
vie
vied
view
viewdata
viewpoint
vigil
vigilance
vigilant
vigorous
vigour
vilified

Vv

vilify
vilifying
villa
village
villi
villous
villus
viloxazine
vinblastine
vinca
vinca alkaloid
Vincent's angina
vincristine
vinculum
vindesine
vindicate
vindicated
vindicating
vindictive
vinegar
vintage
vinyl
Vioform-Hydro·
  cortisone®
violate
violated
violating
violation
violence
violent
viper
viraemia
viraemic
viral
virgin
virginity
viricidal
viricide
virile
virilising
virilism
virility

virion
virologist
virology
virtual
virtually
virtue
virtuosity
virtuous
virulence
virulent
virus
viruses
visa
visas
vis-à-vis
viscera
visceral
visceroptosis
viscid
viscose
viscosity
viscous
viscus
visibility
visible
visibly
vision
visit
visitor
Viskaldix®
visor
vista
visual
visualization
visualize
visualized
visualizing
visually
vital
vital capacity
vitality
vitally

vitalograph
vitamin
vitamin A
vitamin B
vitamin B_1
vitamin B_2
vitamin B_6
vitamin B_{12}
vitamin C
vitamin D
vitamin E
vitamin K
vitiligo
vitreous
vitreous humor
vitriol
vivacious
vivacity
viva voce
vivid
vividness
vivisection
viz
vocabularies
vocabulary
vocal
vocal chord
vocal fremitus
vocalis muscle
vocally
vocation
vocational
vociferous
voice
voiced
voicing
void
volatile
volition
volitional
Volkmann's ischaemic
  contracture

volt
voltage
Voltarol®
volte-face
volume
volumetric
voluminous
voluntarily
voluntary
volunteer
volvulus
vomer
vomit
vomited
vomiting
vomitus
von Gierke's disease
von Recklinghausen's
  disease
von Willebrand's
  disease
vortex
vortexes
vortices
vote
voted
voting
vouch
voucher
vow
vowel
vox
voyage
voyaged
voyaging
voyeur
voyeurism
vulgar
vulgarity
vulnerability
vulnerable

vulsella
vulsellum
vulva
vulval
vulvar
vulvectomy
vulvitis
vulvovaginal
vulvovaginitis
vying

Ww

wad
wadding
wade
waded
wading
wafer
wage
waged
waggon
waging
wail
waist
wait
waiter
waiting-room
waitress
waive
waived
waiving
wake
waked
wakeful
waken
wakened
waking

Waldenström's
  purpura
  hyperglobulinaemia
walkie-talkie
Wallerian
  degeneration
wallet
wallpaper
walnut
wan
wander
wanderer
wane
waned
waning
want
ward
warden
warder
wardrobe
ware
warehouse
warfarin
warily
warm
warmth
warn
warp
warrant
warranty
warrior
warship
wart
wary
was
wash
wash-hand basin
Wasserman test
wastage
waste
wasted
wasteful

wastepaper
wasting
watch
watches
watchful
watchman
watchmen
water
water-borne
waterbrash
waterfall
Waterhouse-
  Friderichsen
  syndrome
waterlogged
waterproof
watery
watt
wattage
wave
waved
wave-form
wavelength
waver
waving
wavy
wax
waxy
wayward
weak
weaken
weakling
weakly
weakness
weal
wealth
wealthier
wealthiest
wealthy
wean
weaned
weaning

weapon
wear
wearable
wearer
wearied
wearily
wearing
wearisome
weary
wearying
weather
weatherbeaten
weave
weaving
web
webbed
webbing
Weber's test
Wechsler-Bellevue
  test
we'd
wedge
wedged
wedging
Wednesday
week
weekday
weekend
weekly
weep
weeping
weigh
weighed
weighing
weight
weighty
Weil-Felix test
Weil's disease
weir
weird
welcome
welcomed

welcoming
welfare
we'll
well
Welldorm®
wellingtons
well-off
well-to-do
welt
welter
Wenckebach
  phenomenon
went
wept
we're
were
weren't
Wernicke's
  encephalopathy
Wertheim's
  hysterectomy
west
Westergren method
westerly
western
westward
westwards
wet
wetness
wetter
wettest
wetting
we've
wharf
wharfs
Wharton's jelly
wharves
what
whatever
whatsoever
wheel
wheelchair

wheeze
wheezed
wheezing
when
whenever
where
whereabouts
whereas
wherefore
whereupon
wherever
wherewithal
whet
whether
whetted
whetting
which
whichever
whiff
while
whilst
whim
whiplash
Whipple's disease
whipworm
whisker
whiskies
whisky
whisper
whispering
  pectoriloquy
whistle
whistled
whistling
Whit
white
white-collar worker
whiten
whiteness
whitewash
Whitfield's ointment
whitlow

Whitsun
who
whoever
whole
wholesale
wholesaler
wholesome
who'll
wholly
whom
whoop
whooping cough
whorl
whose
why
wicked
wickedness
wicker
Wickham's striae
Widal test
wide
widely
widen
widened
widening
widespread
widow
widower
width
wield
wife
wild
wilderness
wildness
wile
wilful
wilfully
will
willed
willing
Wilm's tumour
Wilson's disease

wily
win
wince
winced
winch
winches
wincing
wind
winded
windfall
winding
winding-up
window
windscreen
windy
winning
winter
wintergreen
Wintrobe haematocrit
  or tube
wintry
wipe
wiped
wiper
wiping
wire
wired
wireless
wiring
wiry
wisdom
wise
wish
wishbone
wishes
witch hazel
withdraw
withdrawal
withdrawing
withdrawn
withdrew
wither

Xx

withheld
withhold
withholding
within
without
withstand
withstanding
withstood
witness
witnesses
witticism
wittily
witty
wives
wizened
wobble
wobbled
wobbling
wobbly
woke
woken
Wolff-Parkinson-White
  syndrome
woman
womanly
womb
women
won
wonder
wonderful
wonderfully
won't
wooden
woodland
Wood's light
woodwork
wool
woollen
woolly
word
wording
wore

workable
worker
workman
workmanship
workmen
world
worldly
worm
worn
worried
worries
worry
worrying
worse
worsen
worship
worshipped
worshipping
worst
worth
worthily
worthless
worthy
would
would-be
wound
wove
woven
wrap
wrapped
wrapper
wrapping
wrath
wreak
wreath
wreathe
wreathed
wreathing
wreck
wreckage
wrecked
wrecking

wretched
wriggle
wriggled
wriggling
Wrigley's forceps
wring
wringing
wrinkle
wrinkled
wrinkling
wrist
writ
write
writhe
writhed
writhing
writing
written
wrong
wrongful
wrongfully
wrote
wrought-iron
wrung
wry
wry-neck
Wuchereria
Wuchereria bancrofti
Wysoy®

Xx

xamoterol
xanthelasma
xanthine
xanthine-oxidase
xanthinuria
xanthochromia

xanthochromic
xanthoma
xanthomata
xanthosis
xenon
xenophobia
Xenopsylla
xeroderma
xerophthalmia
xerosis
xerostomia
Xerox®
xipamide
xiphisternal
xiphisternum
xiphoid
X-Prep®
X-ray
X-rayed
X-raying
xylene
Xylocaine®
xylometazoline
Xyloproct®
xylose

Yy

yacht
yachting
yachtsman
yard
yardstick
yarn
yawn
yaws
year
yearly

yearn
yeast
yell
yellow
yellow fever
yelp
yes
yesses
yesterday
yield
yoga
yoghourt
yolk
you'd
you'll
young
youngster
your
you're
yourselves
youth
youthful
youthfully
you've
yttrium
Yugoslavian
Yutopar®

Zz

Zaditen®
Zagreb antivenom
Zantac®
Zarontin®
zeal
zealot
zealous
zenith

zero
zest
Zestril®
zidovudine
Ziehl-Nielsen method
or stain
zigzag
zigzagged
zigzagging
zimmer
zinc
zip
zipped
zipping
zodiac
Zoladex®
Zollinger-Ellison
syndrome
zona
zona pellucida
zone
zoning
zoological
zoologist
zoology
zoonoses
zoonosis
zoster
Zovirax®
Z-plasty
zuclopenthixol
zygoma
zygomatic
zygote
Zyloric®

Appendices

Degrees, diplomas and qualifications

BA	Bachelor of Arts
BC	Bachelor of Surgery
BCh	Bachelor of Surgery
BChD	Bachelor of Dental Surgery
BChir	Bachelor of Surgery
BDS	Bachelor of Dental Surgery
BDSc	Bachelor of Dental Science
BHyg	Bachelor of Hygiene
BM	Bachelor of Medicine
BMedSc	Bachelor of Medical Science
BN	Bachelor of Nursing
BSChB	Bachelor of Surgery
BSc	Bachelor of Science
CBE	Commander of the Order of the British Empire
ChB	Bachelor of Surgery
ChD	Doctor of Surgery
ChM	Master of Surgery
CIH	Certificate in Industrial Health
CMChM	Master of Surgery
CNO	Chief Nursing Officer
DA	Diploma in Anaesthetics
DAP&E	Diploma in Applied Parasitology and Entomology
DAvMed	Diploma in Aviation Medicine
DBE	Dame Commander of the Order of the British Empire
DBO	Diploma of the British Orthoptic Council
DCh	Doctor of Surgery
DCH	Diploma in Child Health
DChD	Doctor of Dental Surgery
DCM	Diploma in Community Medicine
DCMT	Diploma in Clinical Medicine of the Tropics
DCP	Diploma in Clinical Pathology
DCPath	Diploma of the College of Pathologists
DCR	Diploma of the College of Radiographers
DDO	Diploma in Dental Orthopaedics
DDR	Diploma in Diagnostic Radiology
DDS	Doctor of Dental Surgery
DFHom	Diploma of the Faculty of Homeopathy
DIH	Diploma in Industrial Health
DipED	Diploma in Education
DM	Doctor of Medicine
DMD	Doctor of Dental Medicine
DMR	Diploma in Medical Radiology
DMRD	Diploma in Medical Radiodiagnosis

DMRT	Diploma in Medical Radiotherapy
DO	Diploma in Opthalmology
DObstRCOG	Diploma of the Royal College of Obstetrics and Gynaecology
DOrth	Diploma in Orthodontics
DOMS	Diploma in Opthalmic Medicine and Surgery
DPD	Diploma in Public Dentistry
DPH	Diploma in Public Health
DPhil	Doctor of Philosophy
DPhysMed	Diploma in Physical Medicine
DPM	Diploma in Psychological Medicine
DR	Diploma in Radiology
DRCOG	Diploma of the Royal College of Obstetricians and Gynaecologists
DRCPath	Diploma of the Royal College of Pathologists
DRM	Diploma in Radiation Medicine
DS	Doctor of Surgery
DSc	Doctor of Science
DSM	Diploma in Social Medicine
DTM	Diploma in Tropical Medicine
DTMH	Diploma in Tropical Medicine and Hygiene
EN	Enrolled Nurse
FCSP	Fellow of the Chartered Society of Physiotherapists
FDS	Fellow in Dental Surgery
FFARCS	Fellow of the Faculty of Anaesthetists of the Royal College of Surgeons
FFCM	Fellow of the Faculty of Community Medicine
FFCMI	Fellow of the Faculty of Community Medicine in Ireland
FFD	Fellow of the Faculty of Dental Surgeons
FFDRCS	Fellow of the Faculty of Dental Surgery of the Royal College of Surgeons
FFHom	Fellow of the Faculty of Homeopathy
FFR	Fellow of the Faculty of Radiologists
FLS	Fellow of the Linnean Society
FPCert	Family Planning Certificate
FPS	Fellow of the Pharmaceutical Society
FRACDS	Fellow of the Royal Australasian College of Dental Surgery
FRACGP	Fellow of the Royal Australian College of General Practitioners
FRACO	Fellow of the Royal Australasian College of Ophthalmologists
FRACP	Fellow of the Royal Australasian College of Physicians
FRACR	Fellow of the Royal Australasian College of Radiologists
FRACS	Fellow of the Royal Australasian College of Surgeons
FRANZCP	Fellow of the Royal Australian and New Zealand College of Psychiatrists
FRCD	Fellow of the Royal College of Dentists
FRCGP	Fellow of the Royal College of General Practitioners
FRCOG	Fellow of the Royal College of Obstetricians and Gynaecologists
FRCP	Fellow of the Royal College of Physicians

FRCPath	Fellow of the Royal College of Pathologists
FRCPC	Fellow of the Royal College of Physicians of Canada
FRCPE	Fellow of the Royal College of Physicians of Edinburgh
FRCPI	Fellow of the Royal College of Physicians of Ireland
FRCPsych	Fellow of the Royal College of Psychiatrists
FRCR	Fellow of the Royal College of Radiologists
FRCS	Fellow of the Royal College of Surgeons
FRCSC	Fellow of the Royal College of Surgeons of Canada
FRCSE	Fellow of the Royal College of Surgeons of Edinburgh
FRCSI	Fellow of the Royal College of Surgeons of Ireland
FRIPHH	Fellow of the Royal Institute of Public Health and Hygiene
FRS	Fellow of the Royal Society
FRSH	Fellow of the Royal Society of Health
FRSM	Fellow of the Royal Society of Medicine
FSR	Fellow of the Society of Radiographers
LLB	Bachelor of Laws
LLD	Doctor of Laws
LRCP	Licentiate of the Royal College of Physicians
LRCPI	Licentiate of the Royal College of Physicians of Ireland
LRCS	Licentiate of the Royal College of Surgeons
LRCSI	Licentiate of the Royal College of Surgeons of Ireland
LRFPS	Licentiate of the Royal Faculty of Physicians and Surgeons
MA	Master of Arts
MB	Bachelor of Medicine
MBBS	Bachelor of Medicine, Bachelor of Surgery
MBChB	Bachelor of Medicine, Bachelor of Surgery
MBE	Member of the Order of the British Empire
MC	Master of Surgery
MCh	Master of Surgery
MChir	Master of Surgery
MChD	Master of Dental Surgery
MChOrth	Master of Orthopaedic Surgery
MChOtol	Master of Otology
MCSP	Member of the Chartered Society of Physiotherapists
MD	Doctor of Medicine
MDD	Doctor of Dental Medicine
MDS	Master of Dental Surgery
MDSc	Master of Dental Science
MFCM	Member of the Faculty of Community Medicine
MFHom	Member of the Faculty of Homeopathy
MFOM	Member of the Faculty of Occupational Medicine
MIBiol	Member of the Institute of Biology
MIH	Master of Industrial Health
MPhil	Master of Philosophy
MPS	Member of the Pharmaceutical Society
MRACGP	Member of the Royal Australasian College of General Practitioners

MRACP	Member of the Royal Australasian College of Physicians
MRACR	Member of the Royal Australasian College of Radiologists
MRad	Master of Radiology
MRANZCP	Member of the Royal Australian and New Zealand College of Psychiatrists
MRCGP	Member of the Royal College of General Practitioners
MRCOG	Member of the Royal College of Obstetricians and Gynaecologists
MRCP	Member of the Royal College of Physicians
MRCPath	Member of the Royal College of Pathologists
MRCPsych	Member of the Royal College of Psychiatrists
MS	Master of Surgery
MSc	Master of Science
MSR	Member of the Society of Radiographers
OBE	Order of the British Empire
PhD	Doctor of Philosophy
RADC	Royal Army Dental Corps
RAMC	Royal Army Medical Corps
RCNT	Registered Clinical Nurse Teacher
RGN	Registered General Nurse
RHV	Registered Health Visitor
RM	Registered Midwife
RMN	Registered Mental Nurse
RN	Registered Nurse
RNT	Registered Nurse Tutor
RSCN	Registered Sick Children's Nurse
SCM	State Certified Midwife
SEN	State Enrolled Nurse
SRN	State Registered Nurse

Commonly used units of measurement and how to type them

name	symbol	name	symbol
ampere	amp	mole	mol
hertz	Hz	newton	N
hour	hr	ohm	Ω
joule	J	pascal	Pa
kelvin	K	second	s
kilogram	kg	unit	u
litre	l	volt	V
metre	m	watt	W
minute	min		

Decimal prefixes may be combined with the above units:

prefix	symbol	meaning	combination	symbol
deci-	d	one tenth of	decilitre	dl
centi-	c	one hundredth of	centilitre	cm
milli-	m	one thousandth of	millimole	mmol
micro-	μ	one millionth of	microgram	μg
nano-	n	10^{-9}	nanogram	ng
pico-	p	10^{-12}	picogram	pg
milo-	k	one thousand times	kilometre	km
mega-	M	one million times	megavolt	MV

Combination units may be written in symbol form as shown in the following examples:

millimoles per litre	mmol/l
milligrams per kilogram	mg/kg
units per litre	u/l

Common abbreviations

This list contains abbreviations, some of which are often and some of which are always retained, rather than typed out in full:

AA	Alcoholics Anonymous
ACBS	Advisory Committee on Borderline Substances
ACTH	adrenocorticotrophic hormone
ADH	anti-diuretic hormone
AFP	alphafetoprotein
AID	acquired immune deficiency syndrome
AIH	artificial insemination by husband
ARC	AIDS-related complex
ASD	atrial septic defect
ASO	antistreptolysin O
AV	arteriovenous
AV	atrioventricular
AZT	azidothymidine
B.C.G.	Bacille-Calmette-Guérin
b.d.	*bis die* (twice a day)
BMA	British Medical Association
BMJ	British Medical Journal
BNF	British National Formulary
BP	blood pressure
°C	degrees Celsius (or centigrade)
CAPD	continuous ambulatory peritoneal dialysis
CAPE	Clifton Assessment Procedures for the Elderly
CAT	computerized axial tomography
CDH	congenital dislocation of the hip
CMV	cytomegalovirus
CNS	central nervous system
c/o	care of
CPK	creatine phosphokinase
CSF	cerebrospinal fluid
CSSD	Central Sterile Supplies Department
CT	computerized tomography
CTG	cardiotocograph
CV	curriculum vitae
CVA	cerebrovascular accident
D&C	dilatation and curettage
DHSS	Department of Health and Social Security
DNA	Disablement Resettlement Officer
DVT	deep venous thrombosis
ECG	electrocardiogram
ECT	electroconvulsive therapy

EDC	expected date of confinement
EDD	expected date of delivery
EEC	European Economic Community
EEG	electro-encephalogram
ELISA	enzyme-linked immunosorbent assay
EMG	electromyogram
ENT	ear, nose and throat
ERCP	endoscopic retrograde cholangio-pancreatography
ESR	erythrocyte sedimentation rate
etc	*et cetera* (and so on)
°F	degrees Fahrenheit
FEV	forced expiratory volume
FPA	Family Planning Association
FSH	follicle-stimulating hormone
GCFT	gonococcal complement fixation test
GIFT	gamete intra-fallopian transfer
GMC	General Medical Council
GNC	General Nursing Council
GP	General Practitioner
GTN	glyceryl trinitrate
Hb	haemoglobin
HCG	human chorionic gonadotrophin
HIV	human immunodeficiency virus
HMSO	Her Majesty's Stationery Office
Ig	immunoglobulin
IQ	intelligence quotient
IUD	intra-uterine contraceptive device
IV	intravenous
IVF	in vitro fertilization
IVP	intravenous pyelogram
IVU	intravenous urogram
LATS	long-acting thyroid stimulator
LH	luteinizing hormone
LMC	Local Medical Committee
LMP	last menstrual period
LSD	lysergic acid diethylamide
MCV	mean corpuscular volume
MMR	mumps, measles and rubella
MRC	Medical Research Council
MSC	Manpower Services Commission
NHS	National Health Service
NMR	nuclear magnetic resonance
NSAID	non-steroidal anti-inflammatory drug
NSU	non-specific urethritis
PAYE	Pay As You Earn

PMS	premenstrual syndrome
pp	*per procurationem* (for, on behalf of)
PR	*per rectum*
prn	*pro re nata* (when required)
PUO	pyrexia of unknown origin
PUVA	psoralens with ultraviolet light (UV-A)
PV	*per vaginam*
q.i.d.	*quater in die* (four times a day)
qv	*quod vide* (which see)
RAST	radioallergosorbent test
RDS	respiratory distress syndrome
re	with reference to
REM	rapid eye movement
Rh	Rhesus factor
RNA	ribonucleic acid
RSV	respiratory syncytial virus
SLE	systemic lupus erythematosus
T_3	triiodothyronine
T_4	thyroxine
t.d.s.	*ter die sumendum* (three times a day)
TIA	transient ischaemic attack
t.i.d.	*ter in die* (three times a day)
TSH	thyroid-stimulating hormone
UV	ultraviolet
VAT	value added tax
VDRL	Veneral Disease Reference Laboratory
VDU	visual display unit
vis	*videlicet* (namely)
VSD	ventricular septal defect
WBC	white blood count
WHO	World Health Organization
wpm	words per minute